The Diet Denominator:
Fill Your Tank 1

A Practical Guide to Choosing Low   *s*

Frank G. Bottone, Jr., Ph.D.

Complete with a unique, easy to use food evaluation tool.
With The Diet Denominator, you can "Fill Your Tank for Less" by selecting
foods that are energy lean. As a result, you will fill up on fewer calories,
select smarter foods that you still enjoy, and fell less hungry afterwards.

www.DietDenominator.com

Published by Scriptorium Medica Medical Writing, Inc

A medical writing and publishing company

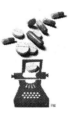

www.ScriptoriumMedica.com

Distributed by Atlas Books

www.AtlasBooks.com

Library of Congress Cataloging-in-Publication Data

Bottone, Jr., Frank G.

The Diet Denominator: Fill Your Tank for Less

A Practical Guide to Choosing Low Energy Density Foods

Diet – Health – Nutrition

ISBN-13: 978-0-615-29422-3

ISBN-10: 0-61529-422-7

Library of Congress Control Number: 2009904205

Published by Scriptorium Medica Medical Writing, Inc

A Medical Writing and Publishing Company

Morrisville, NC

www.ScriptoriumMedica.com

Cover design by Scriptorium Medica Medical Writing, Inc

Distributed by Atlas Books

www.AtlasBooks.com

Phone orders or inquiries: 800-266-5564

Printed in the United States of America

What people are saying about *The Diet Denominator*

Kay E. Schlegel-Pratt, M.S., R.D., L.D.N., C.N.S.D., Founder, Essential Nutrition (www.EssentialNutrition.biz), a nutrition counseling practice in Chapel Hill, NC and Nutritionist, Duke University Medical Center, Durham, NC — Foods with high water and/or fiber content and a lower fat content generally have fewer calories when compared weight for weight with foods lower in water and fiber and higher in fat. The former, high volume foods have been used in weight loss eating plans to create more satisfaction on fewer calories. Now, Dr. Bottone has created a simple, convenient tool using two values available on any food label to help people choose foods with a high volume and lower calorie intake, which can be helpful as they strive to reduce calories for weight reduction.

Brenda Alston-Mills, Ph.D., Associate Dean and Director, Office of Organization and Professional Development for Diversity and Pluralism, Michigan State University — *The Diet Denominator: Fill Your Tank for Less* is a wonderful teaching tool that allows you to read information, practice how to do it, and then apply the knowledge to everyday life. Good nutrition is easy and does become habit forming. I applaud Dr. Frank G. Bottone Jr. for his contribution not only to the field of applied nutrition but also for his genuine concern for the common good.

Steven B. Adler, R.N., B.S.N., B.S., Research Coordinator, Duke University Medical Center, Durham, NC — "*The Diet Denominator* provides a user-friendly system for making smart food choices at home or on-the-go and will serve as a helpful resource to anyone wanting to lose some weight, while, in the process, making a life change and improving their health."

Abbreviations: Ph.D. (Doctor of Philosophy); R.N. (Registered Nurse); B.S.N. (Bachelor of Science Nursing); B.S. (Bachelor of Science); B.A. (Bachelor of Arts); M.S. (Master of Science); R.D. (Registered Dietitian); L.D.N. (Licensed Dietitian/Nutritionist); C.N.S.D. (Board Certified Nutrition Support Dietitian).

What Clinical Researchers are Saying about Energy Density Diets

"Since people tend to eat a consistent weight of food, when the Energy Density of the available foods is reduced, energy intake is reduced." Rolls BJ. The relationship between dietary energy density and energy intake. *Physiol Behav.* 2009. Mar 20 [E ahead of print].

"Reducing dietary energy density, particularly by combining increased fruit and vegetable intakes with decreased fat intake, is an effective strategy for managing body weight while controlling hunger." Ello-Martin JA et al. Dietary energy density in the treatment of obesity: a year-long trial comparing 2 weight-loss diets. *Am J Clin Nutr.* 2007. 85(6):1465-77.

"Both large and modest Energy Density reductions were associated with weight loss and improved diet quality." Ledikwe JH et al. Reductions in dietary energy density are associated with weight loss in overweight and obese participants in the PREMIER trial. *Am J Clin Nutr.* 2007 May;85(5):1212-21.

"Children's energy intake is influenced by the Energy Density of foods and beverages served over multiple days. These results strengthen the evidence that reducing the Energy Density of the diet is an effective strategy for moderating children's energy intake." Leahy KE et al. Reducing the energy density of multiple meals decreases the energy intake of preschool-age children. *Am J Clin Nutr.* 2008 Dec;88(6):1459-68.

"To achieve a low-energy-density diet, individuals should be encouraged to eat a variety of fruits and vegetables as well as low-fat/reduced-fat, nutrient-dense, and/or water-rich grains, dairy products, and meats/meat alternatives." Ledikwe JH et al. Low-energy-density diets are associated with high diet quality in adults in the United States. *J Am Diet Assoc.* 2006. 106(8):1172-80.

About the Author

Frank G. Bottone, Jr., B.A, M.S., Ph.D. received his Doctor of Philosophy (Ph.D.) degree in nutrition biochemistry from the interdepartmental program in nutrition at the College of Agricultural and Life Sciences (CALS), North Carolina State University in Raleigh, NC where his research focused on the cancer chemo-preventive effects of dietary compounds in red wine, soy, and garlic, and various pharmaceutical compounds. While at NCSU and as a biologist at the National Institute of Environmental Health Sciences (NIEHS), Dr. Bottone published numerous peer-reviewed journal articles including 5 first author articles in journals such as *The Journal of Biological Chemistry, The Journal of Nutrition, Molecular Cancer Therapeutics, The Journal of Pharmacology and Experimental Therapeutics,* and *Carcinogenesis* and the corresponding author of a cardiovascular drug safety article appearing in *Current Medical Research and Opinion.*

Before receiving his Ph.D. degree, Dr. Bottone graduated with his Master of Science degree in Biology from Old Dominion University, in Norfolk, VA, and his Bachelor of Arts degree in Biology from Virginia Wesleyan College, in Virginia Beach, VA. Dr. Bottone has received numerous awards including the 2006 Distinguished Alumni Award from the VWC Alumni Association, an honor held by fellow alum Bob Valvano. He received the distinguished 2005 Kenneth R. Keller Research Award for excellence in research and the 2005 Nancy G. Pollock Graduate School Dissertation Award for outstanding scholarly research each from North Carolina State University's College of Agriculture and Life Sciences. Over the past 15 years, He has published over a dozen magazine and newspaper articles in such magazines as *Muscle and Fitness* and *Men's Health.* Dr. Bottone originates from Fair Haven, NJ graduating from Rumson-Fair Haven Regional High School.

Previous Works

Dr. Bottone's previous book, a science and nature experiment book for children entitled *The Science of life: Projects and Principles for Beginning Biologists* (ISBN: 1-55652-382-3; http://www.chicagoreviewpress.com) published by Chicago Review Press, was named to *Smithsonian Magazine's* Notable Books for Children, 2001.

- Kathleen Burke, *Smithsonian Magazine,* November 2001. "At once a lively introduction to the scientific method and a survey of hands-on experiments, this outstanding overview touches on important concepts in botany, bacteriology, molecular biology, mycology, microbiology and more."
- *Science News,* January 19, 2002, "In all, this is a serious but enjoyable book that illustrates the subtle ways in which biology affects our lives every day."
- *Today's Librarian,* book reviews, June 2001, p41: "Bottone's straightforward style is great for young people serious about science. The chapters are easy to understand but introduce solid scientific concepts with terminology."
- Cindy Jones, appearing in *The Bloomsbury Review* magazine, December 2001, p26: "The Science of Life provides 24 well-explained, interesting, biological science fair projects..." "The language in The Science of Life is very easy to understand without being oversimplified."
- Pamela Longbrake, Librarian, Sellers Middle School, Garland, TX, appearing in *The Book Report,* December 2001, p82: "What makes this a better than average book is that the author has anticipated some of the problems young experimenters may have and gives practical suggestions on how to avoid them."
- Maren Ostergard, Bellevue Regional Library, appearing in *School Library Journal* magazine, November 2001: "While the activities are fascinating and educational, some of the items may be difficult to track down, so Bottone has provided a list of suppliers. The volume provides a thorough introduction to this area of science and would be useful in most collections."

Acknowledgements

I would like to thank David Lincoln, M.B.A. for his motivational and challenging discussions regarding the topics discussed in this book. These were instrumental in my decision to take on this challenge.

Additionally, I would especially like to thank my family for their encouragement, and in particular, my wife Stacy, for supporting me and allowing me to invest the time, energy, and resources needed to take on this and all the other challenges in my life.

Words cannot explain how grateful I am to Dr. Alston-Mills not just for putting forth the time, thought, and energy required to write the foreword to this book, for serving as the co-chair my PhD committee, remaining a part of my life to this day, and for serving the community at large.

Last but not least, appreciated is extended to my mom, Jane, and sister, Monica for their editorial and continuous support. I would also like to thank Mair Downing for her exceptional editorial assistance.

Foreword

Brenda Alston-Mills, Ph.D. *is associate dean and director of the Office of Organization and Professional Development for Diversity and Pluralism within the Michigan State University College of Agriculture and Natural Resources (CANR). She was formerly assistant dean of diversity and professor of animal science in the North Carolina State University College of Agriculture and Life Sciences.*

Good grief, another diet book! I thought that most of the plans regarding weight loss had been exhaustively discussed. I was pleasantly intrigued (though not surprised knowing Frank) to find a well thought out plan of action regarding weight control and health. *The Diet Denominator: Fill Your Tank for Less* is an educational and instructional tool as well as easy to read and to understand.

Often, when I'm in a grocery store madly dashing about to get what I need and to depart with exactly what I need and not more, I do take time to notice other patrons. I find many people staring quizzically at the food labels and I often wonder if they have any clue about what the label actually means. I find that many people read the labels because they were told that it is a good thing to do. Giving them all the benefit of the doubt, after all, I read them too; I often wonder how much of the information do the customers really find useful. *The Diet Denominator: Fill Your Tank for Less* offers explanations as to how the percentages of the daily requirements are derived. The book also describes characteristics of the best foods to eat. Even better, the author points out the two pieces of meaningful information that are necessary to determine *The Diet Denominator*: The serving size and the number of calories.

What and how much people actually eat along with their weight are very private issues. *The Diet Denominator* provides a plan whereby one can set a personal goal that can be used to reflect personal achievement. Thus, the individual is empowered to make an actual assessment of what is eaten and how much is eaten with a mechanism to achieve a realistic plan to decrease food volume and density.

Numbers, the dreaded math thing, is another aspect of how this book simplifies the plan. The author provides a step-by-step method of using the two main features on the food label to calculate *The Diet Denominator*. What's more, many of the common foods that we eat are given to us in the tables provided. Again, the book is an educational and instructional tool.

(continued on next page)

My favorite aspect of the book is the idea of keeping a food journal or food diary. Diaries and journals allow us to keep our secrets and to share with others only what we wish. A major benefit is that journals and diaries provide knowledge by connecting the physical act of handwriting or inputting using a keyboard to the visual. Those connections facilitate mental awareness of our actions and habits. We have to be aware of them before we can change them. Once again, journals and diaries provide a means of tracking progress, which, in itself, is an affirmation and reaffirmation of personal success.

Finally, the glossary at the end of the book translates the complex to the simple. Words that are a part of scientific jargon can be confusing to those who are not trained in technical language. The book can be read without intimidation and provides another example of how it can be used to educate.

The Diet Denominator: Fill Your Tank for Less is a wonderful teaching tool that allows you to read information, practice how to do it, and then apply the knowledge to everyday life. Good nutrition is easy and does become habit forming. I applaud Dr. Frank G. Bottone Jr. for his contribution not only to the field of applied nutrition but also for his genuine concern for the common good.

Dr. Brenda Alston-Mills

Author Introduction

The foundation to any good diet plan is a healthy and balanced diet and lifestyle with the hope of making small, incremental improvements in your health and weight over time. This is best achieved by setting very short-term goals and objectives, meeting them, and acknowledging yourself for a job well done. A healthy lifestyle most often consists of moderate exercise, consuming enough fruits and vegetables, limiting alcohol consumption, eating most foods in moderation and eating a low **calorie**[1] diet. A diet based on a healthy lifestyle generally results in weight loss and the ability to keep the weight off over the long-term. For most of us, this is easier said than done.

With *The Diet Denominator*, you can eat fewer calories without feeling hungry. This plan allows you to choose between the foods you enjoy, based on their **energy density**. As a result, you consume fewer calories without eating less food or feeling hungry. If followed correctly, *The Diet Denominator* will serve as an aid to educate and assist you in choosing the right foods based on their energy density. Sometimes this can be obvious, other times it is not so obvious. Following this plan allows you to achieve your weight loss or maintenance goals more easily and effectively.

The Diet Denominator is for those that are practical and feel that their diet should be practical as well. For any diet plan to prove successful, dieters must stick to the plan and be able to apply it to situations typical to their lifestyle. My reccomendation is to choose a diet plan that is simple and easy to understand, and one that you can utilize as part of your daily routine.

This diet plan is unique. No other plan makes use of this food evaluation tool or provides an easier, faster way to make informed food choices. The premise of this book is based on sound science. *The Diet Denominator* uniquely captures the most fundamental scientific principles of nutrition, the calorie and the **gram**, which together determine the energy density, and presents this concept in a way that can be easily understood, followed, and applied to achieve smart weight control that lasts. This plan is intended to work in real-life situations such as at fast food restaurants. This book is based on sound science, yet easy to read and implement as it is not overly scientific or impossible to follow. With that in mind, while reading this book, if you come across terms or concepts that you are not familiar with, be sure to check Appendix 1 in the back of this book to assist you in understanding these points.

---

[1] Refer to Appendix 1: Terms to Learn, for definition of terms indicated in bold throughout this book.

Before You Begin

Now that you have made the decision to lose weight the smart way, with an educational weight loss plan, keep in mind that your chances of success are greater if you incorporate an exercise routine with this or any diet plan.

Before begining this or any diet or weight loss regimen, always consult your physician to ensure you are healthy enough for diet and exercise and that the diet meet your individual needs. It is also recommended that you consult a registered dietitian to discuss your dieting needs.

That said, welcome to *The Diet Denominator: Fill Your Tank for Less.*

Table of Contents

1.   Welcome to *The Diet Denominator: Fill Your Tank for Less* 1

2.   The facts about calories, fats, proteins, and carbohydrates 10

3.   Caloric content, energy density, and volumetric diet plans 17

4.   How is *The Diet Denominator* different from other diets? 22

5.   What is *The Diet Denominator*? 32

6.   Satiety (Feeling of Fullness) 46

7.   Fill Your Tank for Less 55

8.   What is your magic number? 60

9.   How do snack foods measure up to *The Diet Denominator*? 66

10.   How do fast foods measure up to *The Diet Denominator*? 72

11.   How do everyday foods measure up to *The Diet Denominator*? 78

12.   Empty calories and *The Diet Denominator* 83

13.   Understanding food labels and *The Diet Denominator* 86

14.   Keeping the Weight Off 92

15.   Summary 94

      Appendix 1: Terms to Learn 96

      Appendix 2: Diet Denominator Tool 98

      Appendix 3: Diet Denominator of Some Common Food Items 100

      Appendix 4: Diet Denominator of your Favorite Foods 103

      Appendix 5: Weekly Diet Journal 104

1. Welcome to *The Diet Denominator: Fill Your Tank for Less*

The Diet Denominator: Fill Your Tank for Less is a unique new diet plan based on sound science but designed for your hectic lifestyle. This book will provide you with a simple and easy way to learn how to evaluate food options at home, in the grocery store, and even while eating at fast food restaurants so that you can consume fewer calories while choosing foods that you enjoy.

The Diet Denominator: Fill Your Tank for Less is an energy density (**volumetrics**) diet plan with an exciting new twist that makes this plan practical and easy to incorporate into your everyday routine. With *The Diet Denominator*, it is not the amount of food that you eat, but the energy density of the foods that you choose that will enable you to achieve your weight loss or maintenance goals. As a result, with this plan, you can eat the same – or even more – food without gaining weight. The secret is consuming fewer calories while eating foods that make you feel full (discussed in the chapter on satiety).

Thus, with this diet, there are no more fancy diets, special meals, taking potentially unsafe diet pills, or depriving yourself of all the food choices you desire. If you are an adult, parent, adolescent, or teen, this book is sure to help you or a loved one learn how to make informed food choices and become a part of your everyday life because it is easy to follow, implement, and apply no matter what your lifestyle.

This book is designed with you, the dieter, in mind. Importantly, this book is written at a level that is easy to understand while containing bonus sections titled "Did you know?", "Diet Denominator facts", "Take home messages", and "Want to learn more?" ideal for the more advanced reader or for those that want a deeper understanding of the material. This makes it easy for you to distill what you really need to learn from what you will want to learn. Before you are introduced to *The Diet Denominator*, let's start by introducing you to why there is such a need for a completely unique diet plan.

A diet plan that simply limits the types of foods you eat is not enough for today's dieter, in part, because there are too many food items to choose from at home, in grocery stores, and especially at fast food and other restaurants, making it impossible for you to feel satisfied. You may have noticed there has been a rapid increase in the number of diet books. Nevertheless, weight problems and **obesity**[2] have reached epidemic proportions in adults and children. In a recent review article that received some media attention, it was stated that at present, 66% of adults are **overweight** or obese and that by the year 2015, 75% of adult Americans will be

---

[2] Refer to Appendix 1: Terms to Learn, for definition of terms indicated in bold throughout this book.

overweight or obese. [3] This trend has continued over the past few decades despite recent advancements in health and nutrition and shows no signs of slowing down.

The epidemic of overweight and obesity in the United States is further illustrated below using data obtained as part of the Center for Disease Control and Prevention, National Center for Chronic Disease Prevention and Health Promotion, Behavioral Risk Factor Surveillance System (BRFSS) data in Figure 1 and Figure 2. [4]

Figure 1   Prevalence of Overweight in the United States

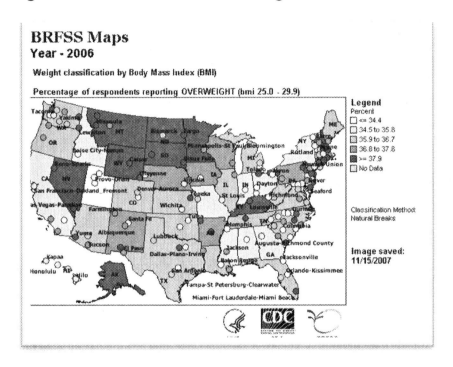

---

[3] Wang Y, Beydoun MA. The obesity epidemic in the United States--gender, age, socioeconomic, racial/ethnic, and geographic characteristics: a systematic review and meta-regression analysis. *Epidemiologic Reviews.* 2007;29:6-28.
[4] Centers for Disease Control and Prevention (CDC). Behavioral Risk Factor Surveillance System Survey Data. Centers for Disease Control and Prevention. 2006.

Figure 2   Prevalence of Obesity in the United States

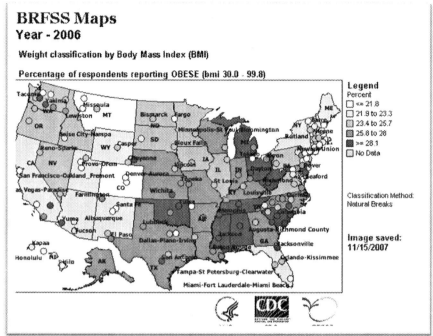

Despite the fact that there are numerous diet plans on the market today, it is clear that something important is missing from those plans because they do not seem to meet the needs of most dieters with overweight and obesity on the rise. Certainly the accessibility of inexpensive and often high caloric value of questionable nutritional value is partly to blame. Combined, these facts indicate that a new diet plan that is backed by science yet easier to understand, implement, and apply to everyday life is needed to make an impact on what might be considered one of the most significant health problems in recent American history.

While overweight and obesity are on the rise, American's fitness levels are decreasing. One measure of fitness is body mass index (BMI). BMI is a tool used to estimate the body composition of individuals using a scale that is easy to use and compare. BMI is on the rise in America. BMI is a ratio of two numbers. It is important to note that potential limits to using the BMI. It may overestimate body fat in athletes with significant muscle mass and may underestimate body fat in the elderly or others who have lost muscle mass. Figure 3 is an illustration indicating the ranges and classifications of BMI, which you can use to calculate your own BMI and track your changes.

Figure 3   Body Mass Index (BMI) Chart

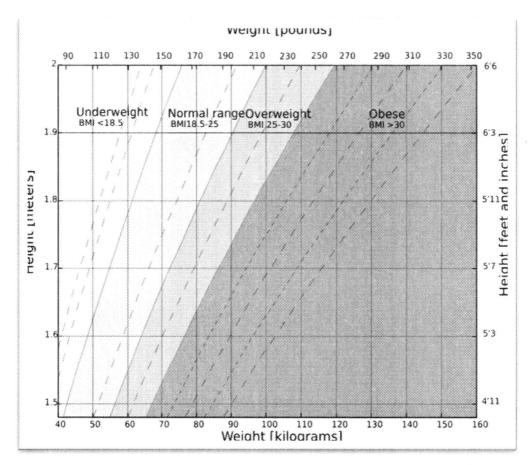

Maintaining a healthy diet and fitness level is important for various reasons. Obesity and type 2 diabetes mellitus (adult-onset diabetes) are closely linked with one another. This means that, when someone is overweight, they are more likely to have diabetes when someone has type 2 diabetes they are more likely to be overweight. In fact obesity is a leading cause of diabetes in the United States. It is no surprise that similar to obesity, diabetes is becoming epidemic in the United States as illustrated using data obtained as part of the Center for Disease Control and Prevention, National Center for Chronic Disease Prevention and Health Promotion, Behavioral Risk Factor Surveillance System (BRFSS) in Figure 4.

Figure 4 Prevalence of Diabetes in the United States

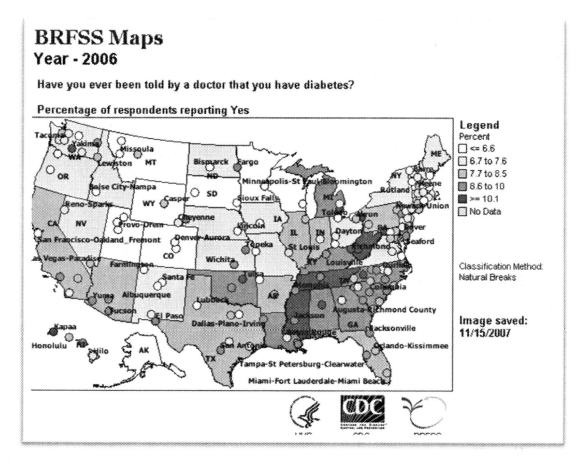

This trend is troubling. In addition to diabetes, obesity is an independent risk factor for other ailments including hypertension (high blood pressure); hypercholesterolemia (high cholesterol); myocardial infarction (heart attack); certain cancers including cancer of the colon, rectum, and prostate in men and of the breast, cervix, endometrium, and ovary in women; obstructive sleep apnea (stop breathing); osteoarthritis and other orthopedic disorders (pertaining to disorders of the skeletal system and associated muscles, joints, and ligaments); infertility; gastroesophageal reflux disease (acid reflux); and urinary stress incontinence (unable to restrain natural discharges or evacuations of urine).

It can only be concluded that as educators, parents, family members, and Americans in general, we are either failing to recognize this as a problem, we are not sufficiently concerned by this problem, or more likely, we have not done a sufficient job of providing appropriate alternatives to prevent this trend from continuing. The question remains; what can be done about it?

Diet Denominator Facts: How is BMI calculated?

BMI is calculated by taking a person's body weight divided by their height squared (body weight / (height x height). Units can be in pounds per feet and inches or kilograms per meters.

You can use an online tool such as http://www.nhlbisupport.com/bmi/bmicalc.htm or http://www.cdc.gov/nccdphp/dnpa/bmi/index.htm and simply type in these values (pounds and feet plus inches) or metric units (kilograms and meters) and your BMI is calculated for you! Either way, your BMI falls into one of the classifications listed below. A BMI above 25.0 indicates that you are overweight and a BMI over 30.0 indicates that you are obese as indicated in the chart below.

Once you are aware of your BMI, you can set goals for yourself to achieve a healthier BMI, over time.

BMI KEY

Below 18.5	Underweight
18.5 - 24.9	Normal
25.0 - 29.9	Overweight
30.0+	Obese

To address these issues while taking advantage of recent scientific and other advancements, various diet plans have become available with mixed success. While many of the newer diet plans are based on good scientific principles, people need more than another diet plan that is overly scientific, impossible to follow, and that comes with a highly restrictive or expensive menu. If you are like most people, you have tried a few different diet plans with mixed success. The one advantage of this trial and error process is that you either will or already have learned that if you do not change your way of thinking and the way you approach eating, you are likely to rebound. Another major pitfall of many other diet plans is that they are not realistic in that they cannot be easily followed or incorporated into your daily routine.

For a diet plan to be effective, it has to be unlike most of what you have tried in the past. An effective plan needs to change the way you approach eating, while still being effective, easy to understand, and follow. In other words, a good plan needs to be simple. Leonardo DaVinci, the renowned painter, sculptor, inventor, and jack of all trades stated "simplicity is the ultimate sophistication". That is a compelling statement that holds true in a vast number of circumstances even today.

For any great idea to be transformed into a practical application it must be simple so that it can make common sense to the most number of people who will use and apply the idea. Meanwhile, it must do so across a variety of circumstances. Ultimately, an effective diet plan has to retrain how you think about and choose food items so that it becomes a part of your daily routine. So how is this possible without being overly complicated or difficult to understand? Well, like most great ideas, the answer must be simple.

Diet fads come and go, but eating right begins with making informed food choices resulting in incremental changes over time. The key to weight loss is good nutrition and the key to good nutrition is education. While many newer diet plans focus on educating the reader about dieting and good nutrition, they often come across as overly scientific, impossible to follow, and lack a true system to use their plan. However, most of us are aware that there is a strong correlation between good health and good nutrition; therefore, education alone isn't enough. This plan will not make you choose fruit over a candy bar; however, it will teach you and give you a tool to allow you to make the right choice when you are not sure which choice is best or otherwise might have made the wrong choice accidentally.

Another factor likely responsible for the out of control weight gain seen across America is portion size, which like the average American's bodyweight has steadily increased over the years. Combined, these facts indicate that a new diet plan based on sound science and that is easier to understand, implement, and apply to your daily routine is needed to make an impact on what might be considered the most significant epidemic in American history.

The Diet Denominator does not overwhelm the reader with scientific facts or jargon. While many other plans come with expensive menus or unrealistic food choices and only apply at home, *The Diet Denominator* makes use of the nutrition facts on all food labels. As a result, this plan is easy to apply to anyone, anywhere, anytime. Best of all, *The Diet Denominator* makes common sense and will work for you because it is simple to use and easy to apply to your daily routine. Best of all, there is no complex food pyramid, point systems, or ready-made meals, which if you are like most of us, are of little help.

On that note, welcome to the revolutionary new diet plan: *The Diet Denominator: Fill Your Tank for Less*. With *The Diet Denominator*, you do not have to memorize what foods high or low energy density, high or low **protein** or contain good or bad **carbohydrates**. In fact, you do not need to concern yourself with proteins, carbohydrates, or **fats** at all as *The Diet Denominator* tool does all the calculating for you. This book will provide you with a clear understanding of basic nutrition and dieting principles as they relate to *The Diet Denominator* so that you are equipped with the information you need to make good food choices. That said, what makes this book so different than all the others on the market today is that *The Diet Denominator* comes with a food evaluation tool (Appendix 2) that makes the food evaluation process simple, yet effective across a vast number of circumstances.

Importantly, this diet plan will not cost the consumer money in expensive food items; rather, it will help you to understand one fundamentally simple principle, the energy density of foods, and provide you with a tool that you can take with you allowing you to take advantage of this principle helping you to lose weight.

After reading this book, you will be able to make informed food choices based on an understanding of the energy density of foods you plan to eat. All you need to do to begin losing weight is learn the calculation and start making informed food choices based on their energy density using this tool. In just minutes, you will be able to apply these few simple steps to your everyday diet at home, while grocery shopping, at work, or at school. Because this plan is unique and practical, you are likely to remember how it works and easily be able to apply it to your ever day life. Most of all, you will be interested to learn *The Diet Denominator* of some of your typical food choices that you will want to avoid as well as those you should have been selecting all along.

With *The Diet Denominator*, you do not have to memorize which foods are better or worse, fattening or sliming, high protein or good carbohydrates. No more guesswork! While you cannot eat whatever you want with this diet plan, you will have the ability to quickly and easily select from foods that you enjoy after examining your food choices using this simple plan. You will quickly learn what foods make better food choices based on *The Diet Denominator* without limiting your food choices or changing your diet drastically like with other plans. This plan simply helps you to limit the less optimal (energy dense) food choices and accentuate the better (energy lean) food choices that you already make. You will be surprised at some of the choices that are better (energy lean) and some that are less optimal (energy dense). Over time, you will spare yourself of countless less optimal (energy dense) food choices and thus countless calories helping you achieve your weight loss goals safely and effectively.

Before you begin, let me explain one thing to you. Throughout this book, you will notice that several key principles are brought to your attention on multiple occasions throughout this book. This reiteration was planned so that those points would stick in the back of your mind and repetition is a great tool for learning. So keep that in mind as you start learning about the concepts in this book.

Take home messages

- Overweight and obesity is becoming epidemic in the United States despite recent scientific advances in health and nutrition
- Obesity is a single risk-factor for a variety of debilatating and potentially fatal illnesses
- There is great need for a diet, educational, or other plan to assist dieters in achieving their weigh-loss goals for the betterment of all Americans
- *The Diet Denominator* is a weight loss plan with you in mind. It is a plan for people of all ages and weight concerns. This plan is based on helping you make informed food choices in practical situations

---

Want to learn more? There are two forms of diabetes, type 1 (early onset) and type 2 (adult onset). Type 2 diabetes usually begins after the age of 40 years and accounts for 90% of diabetes in the U.S. and this number is increasing particularly in children who are overweight and that receive minimal exercise. [5]

---

[5] Wardlaw GM, Kessel MW, Anderson JJB. *Perspectives in nutrition*. 5th ed. Boston: McGraw-Hill; 2002.

2. The facts about calories, fats, proteins, and carbohydrates

Be it in the grocery store, a fast food restaurant, or back at home, the food choices and options presented to us seem endless. Despite this fact, all foods are made up of three major macronutrients: fats, proteins, and carbohydrates. Foods also contain micronutrients: **vitamins** and **minerals**, plus water and **fiber** in varying degrees. It is the proportion of these components that lead to the variability in the amount of calories they contain.

As you will learn, you can take advantage of the natural variety in the foods that you eat so that the proportion of calories from these components benefit you in terms of the number of **calories per gram** the foods you choose contain and thus overall number of calories that you consume. This will assist you in achieving your weight loss goals.

Together, you will begin to develop a better understanding of how the caloric content of the foods that you eat vary greatly and learn how to choose between foods based on the energy density in a manner that you would otherwise not have been able to optimize. Certainly if you eat more of one food than another, there is a good chance you will consume more calories. But when comparing the same amount of two foods, it is the proportion of these macronutrients (and water and fiber) that is responsible for the number of calories it contains. Water does not contain food calories while dietary fiber has a very low **caloric content**, which varies based on the amount of digestible (soluble) fiber. As a result, you will be equipped with the information to recognize and make use of this variety to improve your diet, overall health, and bodyweight. As you will learn, the significance of the water and fiber content of foods cannot be overstated when discussing the energy density of foods.

Let's begin by discussing the importance of the ratio of these items in your food has on your diet. All the foods that we eat contain fats, proteins, and carbohydrates in differing ratios. These are the crucial contributors to the calories we consume. One key to dieting is having an understanding of the contribution of these macronutrients to the caloric content of each food item. Perhaps more importantly, is finding a way to utilize this variety in foods to allow you to choose between foods you otherwise enjoy while selecting foods you enjoy that have fewer calories per given amount or volume of food. *The Diet Denominator* will provide you with a way to quickly and easily discern this information. For now, let's discuss how these components contribute to the calories in the food that you eat.

> *Diet Denominator facts*: The American Heart Association makes various diet and lifestyle recommendations. For example, "Burn more calories than you consume, eat fruits and vegetables, and eat less nutrient-poor foods." This is consistent with this plan, and as you will learn, nutrient poor foods have a high Diet Denominator; therefore, you will be eating a healthier diet with this plan. More information is available at: http://www.americanheart.org/

An adequate amount of the right nutrients in the correct proportions is essential to good nutrition. The body metabolizes nutrients whether insufficient, sufficient, or excessive proportions (or portions). The U.S. Department of Agriculture (USDA) recommends a diet consist of 53% of its calories from carbohydrates, 18% from proteins, and 29% from fats represented graphically in Figure 5.

This recommendation has not changed drastically over time with a recommended 30% of calories from fat in based on the 1995 Dietary Guidelines. [6] However, the availability of food, the readiness of premade foods and fast foods, and the increased energy density particularly of cheap food options (often with less nutritional value) has increased drastically over the past several decades.

---

[6] United States. Dept. of Agriculture., United States. Department of Health and Human Services. *Nutrition and your health: dietary guidelines for Americans*. 4th ed. Washington, D.C.: U.S. Dept. of Agriculture: U.S. Dept. of Health and Human Services; 1995.

Figure 5   FDA Recommended Diet: Calories from Fat, Carbohydrates, and Proteins

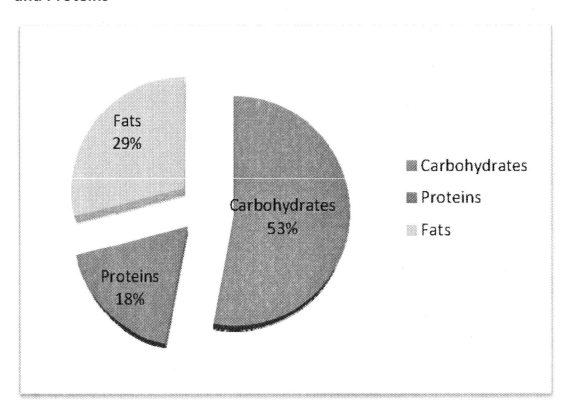

The USDA's recommended proportion of calories from fats, proteins, and carbohydrates is in stark contrast to the average American's diet. The average American diet today is more accurately depicted in the Figure 6. You can see how the proportion of fat in the average diet has increased leading to an increase in calorie consumption. You can also see how many of the common foods that we eat contain a significant amount of calories from fat.

It is important to note, these are not entire meals or daily values, but values from one food item to illustrate how certain food items we eat on a regular basis contribute to the relatively high overall contribution of calories from fat in our diet. These changes in our diets can be explained, in part, because of the availability of food, changes in manufacturing processes, economic pressures, and advances in agriculture. Regardless of the reasons, most Americans and residents of other industrialized nations live in a great time and place where we have ample supplies, access, and availability of food. However, these short term solutions have long term costs to our overall health and well-being.

Figure 6   Typical Diet: Calories from Fat, Carbohydrates, and Proteins

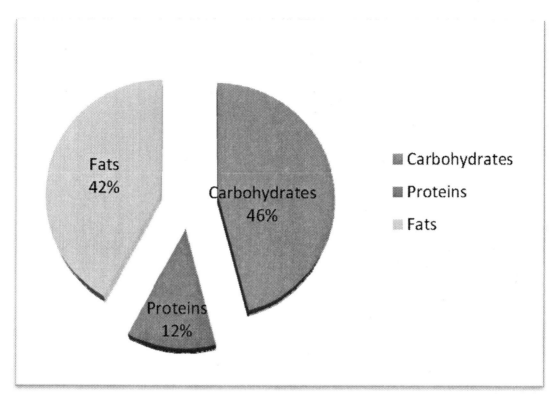

Based on the table below, you can begin to appreciate how a normal diet contains a greater percentage of its calories from fat than is recommended. This is an important point for dieters to understand because fat has 9.0 calories per gram; whereas, carbohydrates and proteins have around 4.0 calories per gram. In other words, the caloric content of fat is roughly twice that of protein and carbohydrates. In addition to fats, carbohydrates, and proteins, foods contain water, fiber, and various micronutrients in differing amounts and proportions. Therefore, another important factor when discussing energy density is the fact that foods with high water and/or fiber content contain fewer calories plus the water and fiber content tends to make you feel full. In this book and elsewhere, foods that contain relatively fewer calories are referred to as energy lean food items; whereas, foods that have more calories are referred to as energy dense food items.

Thus, energy density is the scientific basis of volumetric and similar diet plans. With these plans, you can eat the same amount of food (or even more) so long as the food that you eat has fewer calories and are less energy dense.

Table 1   Calories from Fat, Carbohydrates, and Proteins in Common Foods

Description of Food	Total Calories	Fat Calories, %	Carbohydrate Calories, %	Protein Calories, %
Fried eggs	90	70	4	27
Cream of mushroom soup with water, canned	130	62	28	6
Enchilada	235	61	41	34
Taco	195	51	31	18
Smoked Salmon	150	48	0	48
Tuna Salad	375	46	20	35
Cheeseburger	300	45	37	20
Bacon, egg, cheese, English muffin	360	45	34	20
Beef steak sirloin, broiled, lean	150	36	0	59
Minestrone soup, canned	80	34	55	20
Cheese pizza	290	28	54	21
Refried beans, canned	295	9	69	24

http://www.nal.usda.gov/fnic/foodcomp/Data/

You may be wondering, how to best use this information, because simply trying to avoid fatty foods has not worked in the past. This is an important question, and one that until now has gone unanswered. Since water and fiber contain few calories, they contribute significantly to the variability in the caloric content among various food items by decreasing the overall amount of calories in a given amount of food. An equal amount of some foods naturally contain more energy, whereas others contain less energy.

Table 2   Key Factors Affecting Energy Density of Foods

Item	Effect on *The Diet Denominator*	How it works
Increasing fat content	Increases Diet Denominator	High energy density
Increasing fiber content	Decreased Diet Denominator	Very low energy density (energy lean)
Increasing water content	Decreases Diet Denominator	Zero energy density (energy lean)

It stands to reason that if you eat less fat, you have to eat more protein and/or carbohydrates. Conversely, if you eat food with fewer carbohydrates you have to eat more fat and/or protein. With *The Diet Denominator*, you will learn to make informed food choices resulting in your consuming fewer calories over time.

Diet Denominator Facts: Interested in learning more about the proportions of macronutrients and other components in your food? You can download a free copy of the USDA Guidelines for Americans 2005 from the USDA web site available at:

http://www.health.gov/dietaryguidelines/ [7]

---

[7] United States. Dept. of Agriculture., United States. Department of Health and Human Services. *Nutrition and your health: dietary guidelines for Americans*. 4th ed. Washington, D.C.: U.S. Dept. of Agriculture: U.S. Dept. of Health and Human Services; 1995.

Take home messages

- Foods contain three major macronutrients (constituents), fats, carbohydrates, and protein in varying proportions contributing to the number of calories in any given amount of food
- The variability in macronutrients, water, and fiber all contribute to the energy density of foods
- When the same amount of two foods by weight are compared, the one with the least calories is the most energy lean
- The average diet contains more fat than is recommended by the USDA
- Fats contain more than twice that amount of calories per gram than carbohydrates or proteins
- Water does not contain food calories and fiber is very low in caloric content compared with the three macronutrients
- An adequate amount of the right nutrients in the correct proportions is essential to good nutrition

Want to learn more? Combination Training in Women: Women face different hurtles and objectives when it comes to workout strategies and objectives. But achieving cardiovascular fitness, optimal body composition (% body fat), and favorable blood lipid concentrations (an indicator of overall health) are often desirable to both genders. In an article appearing in the *European Journal of Applied Physiology*, the authors evaluated the effects of resistance, aerobic, and combination training in young, healthy women who trained for 16 weeks followed by 6 weeks of detraining. As a result, only aerobic training resulted in a decrease in triglycerides in the blood and an increase in high-density lipoprotein **cholesterol** (good cholesterol). In addition, aerobic training alone resulted in a 13% reduction in body fat while increasing the participants VO$_2$ maximum (a measure of fitness that determines the volume of oxygen consumed during maximum exercise) by an average of 25%. Strength training and cross training only resulted in improved strength. Therefore, if your objectives are moderate fat loss, cardiovascular fitness, and improved lipid profiles, incorporating an aerobic workout into your routine is likely your best choice. [8]

---

[8] LeMura, LM et al. Lipid and lipoprotein profiles, cardiovascular fitness, body composition, and diet during and after resistance, aerobic and combination training in young women. *Eur J Appl Physiol*. 2000. 82(5-6):451-8.

3. Caloric content, energy density, and volumetric diet plans

With the advent of the internet, there is a wealth of information available on how to diet, what foods to eat, and what foods to avoid. So, why are so many people having weight issues? Making use of all that information, and finding a plan that is right for you is one of the hardest parts about dieting.

Trying to make your way through all the good, bad, and indifferent materials can be difficult. Finding a plan that is easy to use and that you can stick with over the long haul, despite a few ups and downs, is more likely to be successful in keeping track of incremental gains, positive reinforcement, and a sense of purpose all add to the likelihood of success. These are further reasons that a successful diet plan has to be simple to use, easy to follow, and apply to your everyday life.

This chapter serves to introduce you to diet plans based on the energy density of foods. Energy density, also called volumetrics, is a simple yet relatively unfamiliar topic for most people. Energy density is a common principle of nutrition that applies to all types of foods. It is commonly discussed in the animal sciences when talking about animal feed because weight gain is critical in the raising of animals for human consumption; however, it applies to human nutrition especially with regard to losing weight.

Energy density or volumetric diet plans are based on sound science, but until now, have been difficult to implement. This chapter will introduce you to the key concepts in these types of diet plans in the simplest of terms. As you read on, you will find a more detailed explanation of *The Diet Denominator* and what makes it unique, special, and easy to apply to your everyday life.

Volumetric diet plans generally do not make any grand claims or baseless promises nor should they receive the credit when these plans work for you. That is because these plans simply teach you about food and how to make use of the natural variability in terms of the macronutrients in foods and the calories they contain to learn how to select the best food items providing you with a diet plan that you can stick with over the long haul resulting in the positive lifestyle changes that you have wanted.

Most energy density plans require that you learn a great deal about all the foods that you eat and which foods to select and which to avoid. This is easy for some, but overly complex or not practical for most. Therefore, another thing that makes this plan effective is that an understanding or appreciation of the science behind this plan is not necessary for you to be able to use and benefit from *The Diet Denominator* right away.

This plan is easily applied to your dieting routine. In fact, you do not need to understand how it works or memorizing what foods are high or low energy density foods, high protein, or have a low **glycemic index** to apply this plan to your usual eating habits. But first, let's take a look at the basis of this and similar diets.

You may be asking yourself, is it really possible to moderately shift my eating habits and lose weight? The answer is most definitely yes. Some foods have more calories than others on a gram per gram basis. In other words, an equal amount of one food contains more calories than the same amount of another food. What's more, some foods that contain more calories than another do not necessarily taste better, make you feel full, or help keep you feeling full. It stands to reason to lose weight you can eat less food and thus fewer calories. In fact, most other diets require that you simply eat less food be it from a select list of items, premade meals in a box, or by counting calories. What these plans do not take advantage of or even take into consideration is energy density.

The basis of energy density diet plans is that foods vary in their caloric content and this variability can be utilized so that diet goers can consume fewer calories without feeling hungry resulting in weight loss over time. The most important part of such plans is learning how to make the right food choices and being able to do so in real-life situations because these plans work over the long haul, incrementally, over time.

One key to *The Diet Denominator* is that you are able to select food items that are energy lean, thus contain fewer calories, allowing you to eat foods that you desire so long as you are aware that they are energy lean. With this diet plan, there is an easy way to determine which foods are best to select. As a result, you can consume an equal or even a greater volume of food than before while consuming fewer calories, so long as you select foods that are less energy dense. As a result, diet goers can consume the same volume of foods, which contributes to the feeling of fullness much more so than the number of calories. As you will learn, this is different than portion control or calorie counting diet plans, which ultimately aim to reduce the volume of food that you consume but unfortunately leaving you feeling hungry.

So what exactly is energy density? Energy density is a simple principle that deals with the amount of calories (food energy) is in a given amount of food. The energy density of foods can be measured in the number of calories in a given food item per unit of weight (or mass) in grams. Thus, the energy density of foods is measured in calories per gram. You may recall that fat has the highest number of calories per gram thus energy density. The simplest way to eat foods that are less energy dense is to eat foods that contain less fat. However, there are more components of food that contribute to energy density.

Not only does the amount of fat in a food determine the energy density (as opposed to protein or carbohydrates) but the water content and fiber content contribute significantly to the energy density of foods. Water is an important constituent in the foods that we eat. The water content of the foods that we eat varies considerably. Now you may be asking yourself, how is this different than a low calorie diet? Eating a low calorie diet merely recommends that you eat fewer calories, which can be accomplished by limiting the quantity or proportion of fats in the food that you eat. As you probably already know, this becomes increasingly difficult to follow over time. Choosing foods that have a low caloric content or are low in fat is not a realistic way to modify your eating style over the long-term. In part, because choosing those foods items are not that easy. Furthermore, it does not provide you with alternatives. With *The Diet Denominator*, you can choose foods that you enjoy while allowing you to feel full while eating fewer calories.

While this plan is unique, all energy density diet plans are founded on a few simple principles. For example, some foods contain a larger proportion of fats or oils, either naturally (various nuts) or from their preparation (fried foods). Foods with a proportionately high level of fats or oils also have a high caloric content. Many seemingly healthy foods contain high levels of natural fats thus calories and are often energy dense. This is where this plan is so useful because you might not otherwise realize the high energy density of such foods and this tool dose the calculating for you. Conversely, other foods such as soups, many vegetables, and even beans have fewer calories on a gram-for-gram basis, which you may not have realized.

Interestingly, foods that taste good are not necessarily energy dense. Certainly fried foods are energy dense and many people enjoy them; however, when most people have a craving, it is for something salty, sweet, or even something tart. Therefore, with diets based on energy density, you can select food items you enjoy or even crave while sticking to your diet, as long as you choose foods that are energy lean. As a bonus, most of the foods that are less energy dense are healthier; therefore, with this plan, you will begin to eat better while selecting foods that you enjoy without even trying. However, it cannot be overstated that merely knowing that energy lean foods are better for you will not help you to choose energy lean foods in your daily routine on a consistent basis because choosing energy lean foods is not always that easy given some of the food choices we are faced with on a daily basis. That is why this diet plan is different.

As you probably have learned, making the right food choices on the fly, even at fast a food restaurant, is not easy, which is why this plan comes with a food evaluation tool which is simple, easy to learn, and even easier to apply. The evaluation tool is the basis of *The Diet Denominator* and it is simple and easy to use (Appendix 2). Here's how it works. Take the calories per serving and divide that number by the grams per serving, which are listed on any ordinary food label. The resulting number is *The Diet Denominator* and this works for any food item. In other words, this plan is founded on fundamental principles of nutrition, the calorie and the gram; just divide them and compare. Here is an example: The Taco Bell™ Taco Supreme has 200 calories per 113 grams, for a Diet Denominator of 1.7.

Diet Denominator Facts: Heat stress adversely affects your body's ability to burn fat. Instead, your body burns carbohydrates leaving your fat untouched. Thus, you may want to schedule your outdoor exercise when the temperature is comfortable and try to work out indoors when it is hot outside.[9]

---

[9] Febbraio MA. Alterations in energy metabolism during exercise and heat stress. *Sports Med.* 2001;31(1):47-59.

Take home messages

- The basis of energy density diet plans is that foods vary in their caloric content and this variability can be utilized so that diet goers can consume fewer calories resulting in weight loss over time
- Energy density is a simple principle that deals with the amount of food energy in a given amount of food
- The energy density of foods can be measured in the number of calories in a given food item per unit of weight (or mass) in grams
- One key to *The Diet Denominator* is that you are able to select food items that are energy lean, thus contain fewer calories, allowing you to eat foods that you desire so long as they are energy lean

Want to learn more? The simple sugars **glucose**, **fructose**, and **galactose** are the building blocks of disaccharides (meaning two simple **sugars** paired together) and the more complex compounds, polysaccharides (meaning many sugars paired together). Even more complex forms of sugars include the starches, which are digestible and dietary fiber, of which, some are digestible to varying degrees while others are indigestible. Digestible fibers are those that either dissolve or swell in water and are metabolized by bacteria in the large intestine (soluble fiber). Indigestible fibers mostly do not dissolve in water and are not metabolized by bacteria in the small intestine (insoluble fiber). Your body absorbs some of the nutrients, thus calories, from soluble fibers but very little from insoluble fiber. Either way, fiber has a very low energy density and makes a great addition to your diet for this and other reasons. [10]

---

[10] GM Wardlaw and M Kessel. *Perspective in Nutrition.* 5th Ed. p167.

4. How is *The Diet Denominator* different from other diets?

There are a variety of diet books and diet plans on the market today. One simple commonality between familiar diet plans such as the Special K™, Subway™, low fat, meal replacement, and healthful diet plans is that they all unknowingly recommend eating items with a low energy density. In a society where more and more food choices have a high energy density, this often corresponds to a low nutritional value. While many of the newer diet plans are based on educating the reader, another diet plan that is overly scientific, impossible to follow, or that comes with a highly restrictive or expensive menu to achieve your weight loss goals is not needed.

A great plan needs to teach the reader how to make informed food choices and yet be simple, effective, and applicable to almost anyone when selecting foods at home, in the grocery store, or even in a fast food restaurant. Let me introduce you to *The Diet Denominator: Fill Your Tank for Less*. Another thing you may have noticed that many of these plans have in common is that they are overly complicated, too restrictive, filled with scientific jargon, and do not apply to your everyday life. As a result, they do not work over the long haul because they are unrealistic as they do not apply to eating situations outside of your own home.

This plan does not come with outdated pyramids, require you to purchase foods from an expensive menu (then microwave them), or commit to memory what foods you can choose. This plan is not overly restrictive or impractical like many of those plans. *The Diet Denominator*, like some of the other newer diet plans, is an interesting and appealing diet plan that belongs to a class of diet plans known as caloric content, energy density, or volumetric diet plans. However, unless you are a scientist, nutritionist, or want to memorize how much energy is in which foods or want to spend hours searching the internet for recipes then basing your grocery shopping on such a list, other energy density diet plans are not likely useful to you.

If you are someone reading about these plans for the first time, you might wonder what is so special about these plans and how *The Diet Denominator* differs from these plans. This is an easy question to answer. While there are dozens of diet books on the market today; however, these books all lack a practical, quick, and easy to use tool to ensure their success. *The Diet Denominator* consists of a universal, easy to use food evaluation tool that makes dieting simple by allowing the reader to make practical and informed food choices on-the-fly in real time as part of their everyday life.

The Diet Denominator is one of a kind because other diet plans including caloric content, energy density, and volumetric diet plans do not have a universal, easy to use food evaluation tool that you learn easily and that applies to nearly all situations and that you can take with you wherever you go.

So what does a diet plan need to be effective and practical? For a diet plan to be practical, it must apply to your everyday life. The key to dieting is making informed food choices at as many meals as possible, not just in your home or even the grocery store. With *The Diet Denominator* tool, which is the topic of the next chapter, making informed food choices is easy because this tool takes the guesswork, memorization, and complexity out of dieting easy. Best of all, you can use this plan anywhere and at any time, even at a fast food restaurant. While other energy density or volumetric plans are interesting and scientifically valid, they are not practical for use in everyday life.

The Diet Denominator is based on a variety of well-studied, proven scientific principles; however, this diet plan is vastly different than any of the plans on the market today. As you will learn, *The Diet Denominator* is based on sound science and that this plan is not just a theory because you can incorporate this plan into your everyday life. Another advantage of this plan is that it helps you with arguably the most difficult part of any diet, choosing what foods to eat. Often times, dieters such as yourself want to make the right choice but do not even know where to begin or the best foods to choose. Furthermore, over time, eating the same foods becomes boring, expensive, or impractical often causing you to lose interest in the diet.

This book will provide you with the information needed to choose the right foods at home, in the grocery store, or even while eating out simply and easily without preplanned menus, expensive meals, points, pyramids, or other hard to understand and even harder to follow plans. Best of all, once you learn what foods are best to choose, you can begin selecting the foods you enjoy most that fit into the this diet plan. You will be surprised at what foods make better choices according to this plan and what foods you may have thought were good but that should be avoided because of their high energy density. These ideas are expanded upon in the following chapters. Other diet plans simply tell you not to eat snack foods or fast foods, and some might as well say quit eating good tasting food altogether. Because these plans do not apply to many situations they become increasingly complex and hard to follow. Sure, these diet plans would work in a perfect world, if only they were practical and they could tell you what you are supposed to eat. That is, assuming you had the time and money to buy the foods they recommend. However, the truth is that you do not have to eliminate all snack foods or fast food from a healthy weight-loss diet plan and simply selecting what you think are "healthy foods" may not help you achieve your weight loss goals.

So how do you differentiate between those foods you should and should not eat? Most diet plans simply restrict a large subset of foods from your diet, snacks or otherwise. For these plans to apply to almost anyone across a variety of eating habits they have to be highly restrictive. If you want to make a rule that applies to everyone, it has to be grossly generalized making it overly restrictive or inadequate. It is easier for most diet plans to simply state eat fewer calories or don't eat carbohydrates than instruct you as to what foods are good to choose; however, this makes them difficult or impractical to follow. None of these diets provides you with a practical way to implement their plan. In other words, they are impractical. Diet such as these that rely on the dieter to count points continue to buy expensive foods, or to continually select the best foods based on memory are not feasible with these plans. Diet plans that cannot easily be put into action will quickly become nothing more than a fad.

What makes this book unique is that it consists of a rewarding, fun, and easy to use food evaluation tool (Appendix 2) to help you make informed food choices in real time at home, in the grocery store, or even while eating out. The tool is simple, yet you do not have to understand how the tool works to incorporate this plan into your everyday life. Unlike calorie counting or other volumetric diet plans, this plan is simple to use and easy to apply to everyday life. This book is not overly scientific and does not simply categorize foods as good carbohydrates versus bad, low protein versus high or by the number of calories it contains. Using this tool, choosing foods that are less energy dense is easy. For example, you can use this plan wherever you make food choices resulting in your eating fewer calories while feeling full. Best of all, this plan is not overly restrictive, which is one of the leading reasons people are unable to stick to their diets.

With this plan, you are able to consume fewer calories while feeling full without having to study which foods is energy lean or energy dense like with other volumetric (energy density) diet plans, which are overly complex thus difficult to follow. In fact, using this plan, the dieter can select from any foods that they enjoy, so long as they are energy lean, based on *The Diet Denominator*. This book demonstrates in simple terms how you can change your eating habits and make educated food choices quickly and easily in an effort to lose weight more easily and effectively while keeping the weight off. Here is an example so you can see for yourself how easy this plan is to use in your everyday life.

As illustrated in Figure 7, a Kit Kat Bar™ has 286 calories per 55 grams for a Diet Denominator of 5.2.

Calculate The Diet Denominator: Kit Kat Bar™

286 calories / 55 grams = 5.2 on The Diet Denominator scale

Figure 7   Diet Denominator: Sample Calculation

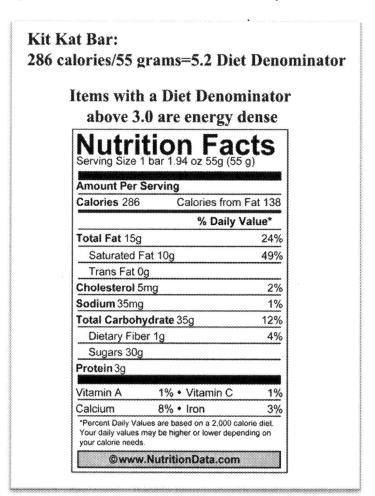

Thus, this snack makes for a less optimal (energy dense) choice. But not all snacks that taste great are energy dense. This plan recommends choosing foods with a Diet Denominator at or below 3.0, or your **magic number** as discussed in that chapter. Thus, as you might imagine, there are many snack items that are recommended over a Kit Kat Bar™ illustrated in this example.

With this plan, all you need is to do this simple math in your head, use a calculator, or use the chart in Appendix 2 to determine *The Diet Denominator* of your food choices to determine which item makes the best choice.

The Diet Denominator is for those that are practical and feel that their diet should be practical, at least if it is to have a chance to be successful. For any diet plan to be successful, the plan must be easy to understand and follow so that the dieter can stick to the diet and be able to apply the diet to situations typical to their lifestyle. One advantage of *The Diet Denominator* is that it can be generalized across a variety of people such as you with a variety of eating habits without being highly restrictive. Over the long term, it is unrealistic to think that a dieter can simply eat less or eat specialized foods or from expensive menus. Even other energy density plans do not have a means to apply their plans. However, it is safe to assume that given an easy method to evaluate food choices on the fly a dieter will make better choices knowing they can choose foods that they like that happen to have fewer calories.

Therefore, with this plan, you are not even on a diet, per se, you are just learning how to choose the right foods time and time again, without memorizing what food items to eat, buying expensive meals or grocery items, or simply restricting your diet so much so that it is not sustainable.

Did you know? A single serving of bananas contains just 200 calories per 225 grams for a Diet Denominator below 1.0 and they are a great source of potassium, which is needed for a healthy heart.

Calculate The Diet Denominator: bananas

200 calories / 225 grams = 0.9 on The Diet Denominator scale

The Diet Denominator is based on some similar principles as energy density or volumetric diet plans. However, *The Diet Denominator* is superior to these types of diets because it provides you with a tangible number you can use to evaluate what foods you should choose simply and easily while in the grocery store, at home, and even at work. The concept of energy density is nothing new and *The Diet Denominator* is more than just another energy density plan. Like most technologies, theories, or inventions, until you can find a practical way to implement them, so that people can actually utilize the plan, they are nothing more than an interesting idea.

The advantage of *The Diet Denominator* is that the idea evolved into a plan that can easily be followed and applied to your hectic lifestyle. What makes *The Diet Denominator* special is that this plan gives you a way to calculate and compare a great variety of foods in real time on the fly in a manner that is simple and easy. Thus, what this plan has that others do not have is a means to assist you in the food evaluation process.

Did you know? There are a variety of diet plans on the market today. If you evaluate some of the better plans using The Diet Denominator scale you will find that these plans conform to this plan. This is an indication that The Diet Denominator can be universally applied across a wide range of situations, foods, and circumstances. For example:

Jared's Subway™ diet™ contains a wide variety of 6-inch Jared sandwiches, each with 6 grams of fat or less. When prepared with wheat bread, lettuce, tomatoes, onions, green peppers, pickles and olives as suggested on their menus, each of these subs score wonderfully according to The Diet Denominator.

Another plan that is useful and can be explained by the principles of The Diet Denominator is the Special K™ diet. The Special K™ diet is a meal replacement diet of sorts. It consists of replacing your regular meals with their foods. In the short term, this can be successful. It is no coincidence that The Diet Denominator of many of their foods is in the recommended range for The Diet Denominator. More information is available at: http://www.specialk.com/

The Diet Denominator works with liquid-based foods as well. For example, the Slim-Fast™ plan is a liquid, meal replacement plan. While this is a liquid meal replacement, this plan still applies just like it applies to soup or other liquid-based foods. Original Slim-Fast™ contains 220 calories per 325 mL [because 1 mL = 1 gram].

Calculate The Diet Denominator: Original Slim-Fast™

220 calories / 325 mL or grams = 0.7 on The Diet Denominator scale

This falls well within the recommended range for The Diet Denominator.

The science behind *The Diet Denominator* is well established and has been understood by many for some time. In fact, there are a few other plans based on energy density. *The Diet Denominator* is the only plan based on an easy to use food evaluation tool to assist you in making informed food choices anytime, anywhere. *The Diet Denominator* gives you a simple formula you can use when looking at any ordinary food label to decide if that food item has an energy density that is part of your diet. As you will learn in Chapter 8 (what is your magic number?), you can customize this plan to fit your goals and desires. Whether you want to lose weight quickly, slowly, or maintain your weight, with *The Diet Denominator*, simply choose a number that is right for you. Alternatively, simply select any food item with a Diet Denominator at or below around 3.0, which is the average Diet Denominator of ordinary food items and begin losing weight. The formula applies to almost all foods, which makes choosing which foods will help you achieve your weight loss (or maintenance) goals simple and easy. *The Diet Denominator* will change the way you make food choices, based first on energy content and then personal preference.

This book will provide you with a fun and easy way to eat the same or even greater volumes of food without gaining weight. This is possible due to the energy density of foods. No more fancy diets, special meals, taking unregulated diet pills, or by depriving oneself of the food choices desired. The details of this plan will be discussed in the coming chapters. For now, here is an example of how you can apply *The Diet Denominator* using a food label from some ordinary food items such as those recommended by Jared of Subway™ sandwiches. Jared's sandwiches are named after their diet plan, which is based off of a man named Jared that made headlines and went on to become their spokesperson after losing a considerable amount of weight after primarily eating meals consisting of a Subway™ sandwich daily for some time. Table 3 illustrates *The Diet Denominator* of some of the Jared's sandwiches.

With *The Diet Denominator*, you can eat more than just sandwiches, but this is a great example of how real food choices can be evaluated with nothing more than a menu using this plan and how the principle of this book was one of the underlying reasons that plan was effective for Jared and many others. Jared and others can evaluate some of the sandwiches that make better (energy lean) choices from Subway™; however, imagine how much easier it would be if you could evaluate nearly all the foods that you are exposed to using *The Diet Denominator*.

Table 3   Diet Denominator of Jared's Recommended Subway™ Sandwiches

6-inch Jared sandwich's*	Food Energy (calories)	Weight (grams)	Diet Denominator
Ham	290	224	1.29
Oven roasted chicken breast	310	238	1.30
Roast beef	290	224	1.29
Subway™ club	320	257	1.25
Sweet onion chicken teriyaki	370	281	1.32
Turkey breast	280	224	1.25
Turkey breast and ham	290	234	1.24
Veggie "delite"	230	167	1.38

*When prepared with wheat bread, lettuce, tomatoes, onions, green peppers, pickles and olives as suggested on their menus.

Other programs have been devised by research scientists that while they are correct in their principles and theories, they lack a way to be useful. Other diet plans based on the energy density of foods (volumetrics), the citric acid cycle (Atkins™ diet), and low **glycemic** foods are great in theory. Many dieters feel that these plans are not easily applied to their lifestyle. Some common diet plans and how they work are illustrated in Table 4.

Table 4   Common Diet Plans on the Market

Types of Diet Plans	How They Work
Atkins™	Low carbohydrate diet
South Beach™	Moderately low carbohydrate diet
Energy Density/Volumetrics	Consume foods that are energy lean
Glycemic Index	Consume foods with a low glycemic index
Weight Watchers™	Portion control
Jenny Craig™	Portion control
Slim Fast™	Meal replacement

Most of these diet plans are highly restrictive. Therefore, you simply run out of enjoyable, realistic, variety in the food choices you can make, and as a result, you will likely begin to stray from the diet. While the volumetric diets on this list provide you with the knowledge to choose the right foods, they do not include an easy to use formula to ensure success, they are rather complex, difficult to understand, and impossible to apply in real world situations. If you spend hours in the grocery store or at home with pad, pencil, and calculator planning and selecting your meals they will work, but who has that time or patience. In other words, those plans are not practical for most people and nearly impossible in the long term for almost all of us.

The Diet Denominator is based on sound science, plus it is so simple that you can use it as a part of your everyday life. In the next chapter, you will learn more the details regarding *The Diet Denominator* and how it can help you achieve your diet goals.

Take home messages

- Caloric content, energy density, and volumetric diet plans are based on sound science and are unique from other diets on the market in that they promote eating fewer calories while eating a sufficient volume of food so that satiety (feeling of fullness) is not compromised
- Energy density diet plans are based on sound science but can be difficult to implement without an easy to use food evaluation tool such as *The Diet Denominator*
- *The Diet Denominator* is vastly different than any of the plans on the market today
- Unlike other diet plans, *The Diet Denominator* is practical and easy to apply to your everyday life

---

Want to learn more? Leptin is a hormone produced by adipose tissue which plays a critical role in the regulation of energy intake, expenditure, appetite, and lipid and carbohydrate metabolism. However, the key function of leptin appears to do with the body's adaptation to reduced energy availability. Leptin is important in obesity and leptin was first discovered in a strain of obese mice. While leptin is thought to reduce appetite, obese individuals seem to have higher circulating levels of leptin, indicating these individuals are resistant to the effects of leptin much like people with type-2 diabetes are resistant to insulin made in their bodies. [11]

---

[11] Havel PJ. *Diabetes*. 53 (Suppl. 1):S143–S151, 2004.

5. What is *The Diet Denominator?*

Despite the fact that there are numerous diet plans on the market today, it is clear that there is something fundamental missing from those plans because they do not seem to meet the needs of most dieters with overweight and obesity on the rise. Certainly the accessibility of inexpensive and often high caloric foods of questionable nutritional value is partly to blame. Combined, these factors might explain why you or someone you know has had difficulty adhering to or maintaining their weight loss goals with any given diet plan. It seems as if these programs were created without the people who follow them in mind. The one thing missing from these plans is convenience.

If dieting was simple and easy to do, you probably would agree that more people would stick more closely to their diet. Traditional (not fad) diet plans are based on a variety of perfectly valid scientific and/or common sense principles such as eating a low calorie diet, low fat diet, portion control, and meal replacement plans. Yet most of you would likely agree that you do not have the time, money, or patience to follow them for the time required to reach your weight loss goals. This is because eating preplanned meals from a cardboard box, eating every meal at home, or preparing two or three meals per day from scratch is not practical given your hectic lifestyle or perhaps even more commonly, you simply cannot afford the meals. In other words, these plans are overly complex and highly restrictive. As a result, they are difficult to follow and over time they become ignored.

Many of the newer diet plans focus on educating you on the importance of a balanced diet, portion control, and maintaining a healthy lifestyle. While these plans attempt to have a long lasting impact by teaching diet goers such as yourself how to eat right, plans such as these are hard to put into practice in everyday life thus they are severely limited. This is because every one of us is constantly being exposed to different food choices on an hour-by-hour, day-to-day, and week-to-week basis. Plus, we each have different eating habits making a "cookie-cutter" diet plan overly restrictive and often impractical, which is why an educational diet plan that allows you to eat regular food items such as this can work even over the long-term. We are all faced with new and unique dieting challenges on a daily basis and need a plan that applies to real-life situations across a variety of circumstances.

The Diet Denominator is a diet plan that is based on the energy density of foods which might sound complex but with this plan, it is actually exceptionally easy to use. With *The Diet Denominator*, you can select foods that are less energy dense quickly and easily using this food evaluation tool (Figure 8).

Calculate The Diet Denominator: sample food label

40 calories / 120 grams = 0.3 on The Diet Denominator scale

Figure 8   Calculate *The Diet Denominator*: Sample Food Label

Nutrition Facts	
Serving Size: 1 cup (120 g)	← *Note the number of grams here.*
Amount per Serving	
Calories 40	← *Note the number of calories here.*
Calories from Fat 0	
% Daily Value *	
Total Fat 0g	0%
Saturated Fat 0g	0%
Monounsaturated Fat 0g	
Polyunsaturated Fat 0g	
Cholesterol 0mg	0%
Sodium 0mg	0%
Potassium 24mg	1%
Total Carbohydrate 29g	10%
Dietary Fiber 1g	4%
Sugars 0.1g	
Protein 4g	8%

The Diet Denominator applies to all situations, all foods, all people, and all types of meals. This is because it is based on a fundamental principle of nutrition, energy density, which is comprised of the calorie and the gram. As you will see, it is not the total fat, **saturated fat**, mono- or poly-**unsaturated fat**, carbohydrates, protein, or even the calories that you should first be concerned with; rather, the energy density of the foods that you select.

You see, all foods contain these items in differing proportions. Simply limiting the number of calories you eat or the amount of fat you eat might work in the short term; however, it is the long-term that matters. The key is being able to choose food items that are energy lean time and time again across a variety of situations.

This plan is not a fad, it is not too good to be true, and you will not see results instantly. What this plan **will do** is give you a tool and teach you how to select energy lean food items time and time again helping you to make informed food choices quickly and easily anywhere you go.

The Diet Denominator is based on the energy density of foods (also known as volumetrics), which is a well tested and proven theory, <u>but until now, lacked a system to use it</u>. Volumetric diet plans require that you make knowledgeable food choices consisting of items that are energy lean, many of which <u>make you feel full</u> and thusly eat less.

With *The Diet Denominator*, you determine if a food item is energy lean or energy dense. The more often you use this plan to assist you with choosing a meal, the better the plan will work and the sooner you can begin losing weight. Unlike calorie counting or other volumetric diet plans, this plan is simple to use and easy to apply to everyday life as it is not restricted to your home.

So what is energy density? The energy density of foods refers to how many calories can be found in any given amount or weight of food. Energy density is a relatively simple concept that has to do with the amount of energy measured in calories contained in a given amount of food and is measured in grams. Energy density plans are often called volumetric diet plans because if you select foods that have a low energy density, you can eat a greater volume (amount) of food while consuming fewer calories. As a result, you are less hungry afterwards, which helps you to lose weight over time.

Using energy density, you can compare foods and categorize them as energy dense versus energy lean foods allowing you to make informed food choices. The more calories in any given amount of food, the more energy dense the food. Energy lean foods have fewer calories per gram than foods that are high in calories. Energy density varies in foods depending on the amount of water, fat, fiber, and nutrients they contain. Certain foods high in fats (deep fried foods) are considered energy dense. Foods that have a low energy density (including those with high water and/or fiber content) are called energy lean.

This plan is flexible. You can select between foods that you like while consuming those that are more energy lean thereby consuming fewer calories or a greater volume of food. By using the unique food evaluation tool, choosing energy lean food items is a snap. Simply choose food items that fall at or below your magic number, which is *The Diet Denominator* of the typical items in your diet, so that you will begin consuming fewer calories. The lower *The Diet Denominator* of the foods you choose, the fewer calories you are going to consume over time thus the more weight you can lose.

The evaluation tool is simple. Divide the calories per serving by the grams per serving (calories/grams) on any food label to obtain *The Diet Denominator*. The highest number on *The Diet Denominator* scale is 9.0 (as all food items have anywhere between 9 calories per gram). Pure fat, butter, and lard have 9.0 calories per grams, and are thus energy dense. The lowest number on *The Diet Denominator* scale is zero, and any foods that fall on this side of the scale are considered energy lean. For example, seltzer water has zero calories per gram. In contrast, carbohydrates and proteins have around 4 calories per gram. Water does not contain calories. Since all foods range from as high as 9 (energy dense) to as low as zero (energy lean) on a scale from energy dense (which you should avoid) to low (which you should select) as shown in Table 5.

You do not necessarily have to pick food items below a certain Diet Denominator, just make modest improvements to your diet based on *The Diet Denominator* of the foods that you select and the results will come over time.

Table 5   Diet Denominator of Major Food Components

Food Group	Diet Denominator (calories per gram)
Protein	4.0
Carbohydrates	4.0
Fats	9.0
Fiber	~2.0
Water	0.0

As you may notice from Table 5, fiber contains a relatively small amount of calories compared with the other food groups. This is but one of the reasons eating a high fiber diet is good for you. Fiber also helps to reduce the absorption of fat and provides roughage good for digestion. Thus, fiber is low in calories, in part, because our bodies do not digest it very well.

More specifically, the amount of calories that your body can utilize from fiber varies based on what percentage of the fiber is digestible (soluble). As a general rule, fiber has less than 2 calories per gram. It is easy to understand that foods with less water have a greater energy density, which is because water has zero calories per gram.

All you have to do is take the food calories on the package, recipe, or menu and divide it by the weight (in grams); there is nothing to buy! That is the basis of *The Diet Denominator*. Yes, it is that simple! With *The Diet Denominator*, you can quickly and easily calculate the energy density of food items allowing you to choose the items that are good, better, or best for you. It is all about awareness and making incremental improvements over time. On average, *The Diet Denominator* of home-cooked foods is around 3. Fast foods generally higher on *The Diet Denominator* scale resulting in the intake of more calories than you need leading to weight gain or, at the very least, an inability to lose weight.

Best of all, with *The Diet Denominator*, if you feel the need to waiver from your diet plan or have a limited number of good food choices at any given meal or food purchase, simply select a food item that is as close as possible to a Diet Denominator of 3 so that you do not blow your plan. Dieting is all about moderation and making informed food choices. It is best to approach dieting one meal at a time. *The Diet Denominator* holds true for any food item, the more energy dense, the higher on *The Diet Denominator* scale the food items will fall and the more calories (per gram) it contains (Figure 9).

Figure 9   ***The Diet Denominator* Scale**

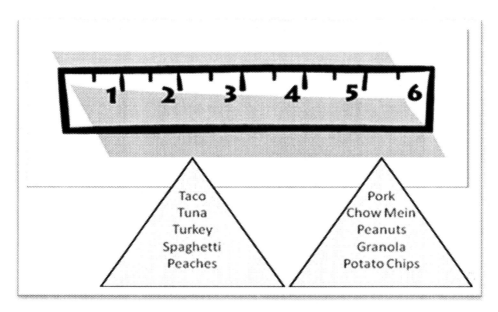

With this plan, you can eat the same volume of food while consuming fewer calories thus still feeling full unlike most diet plans. That is because you will be consuming less energy dense foods. The average Diet Denominator of the ordinary food items prepared from items from the grocery store is around 3.0 and to lose weight, you want to try and choose foods with a Diet Denominator at or below this number or below your magic number as discussed in that chapter.

Keep in mind, this number can be much higher for restaurants, fast foods, and other foods, which is why this plan is so useful. This plan is so simple and easy to use you can make the calculation on your own. As illustrated in Figure 10 and in Appendix 2.

Figure 10   Diet Denominator Tool

Step 1: Start here. Begin by finding the CALORIES of your food item from top to bottom.
Step 2: Find the GRAMS from left to right across the page here.
The number at that intersection is The Diet Denominator.

	50	75	100	125	150	175	200	225	250
50	1	0.7	0.5	0.4	0.3	0.3	0.3	0.2	0.2
75	1.5	1	0.8	0.6	0.5	0.4	0.4	0.3	0.3
100	2	1.3	1	0.8	0.7	0.6	0.5	0.4	0.4
125	2.5	1.7	1.3	1	0.8	0.7	0.6	0.6	0.5
150	3	2	1.5	1.2	1	0.9	0.8	0.7	0.6
175	3.5	2.3	1.8	1.4	1.2	1	0.9	0.8	0.7
200	4	2.7	2	1.6	1.3	1.1	1	0.9	0.8
225	4.5	3	2.3	1.8	1.5	1.3	1.1	1	0.9
250	5	3.3	2.5	2	1.7	1.4	1.3	1.1	1
275	5.5	3.7	2.8	2.2	1.8	1.6	1.4	1.2	1.1
300	6	4	3	2.4	2	1.7	1.5	1.3	1.2
325	6.5	4.3	3.3	2.6	2.2	1.9	1.6	1.4	1.3
350	7	4.7	3.5	2.8	2.3	2	1.8	1.6	1.4
375	7.5	5	3.8	3	2.5	2.1	1.9	1.7	1.5
400	8	5.3	4	3.2	2.7	2.3	2	1.8	1.6
425	8.5	5.7	4.3	3.4	2.8	2.4	2.1	1.9	1.7
450	9	6	4.5	3.6	3	2.6	2.3	2	1.8
475	-	6.3	4.8	3.8	3.2	2.7	2.4	2.1	1.9
500	-	6.7	5	4	3.3	2.9	2.5	2.2	2
525	-	7	5.3	4.2	3.5	3	2.6	2.3	2.1
550	-	7.3	5.5	4.4	3.7	3.1	2.8	2.4	2.2
575	-	7.7	5.8	4.6	3.8	3.3	2.9	2.6	2.3
600	-	8	6	4.8	4	3.4	3	2.7	2.4
625	-	8.3	6.3	5	4.2	3.6	3.1	2.8	2.5
650	-	8.7	6.5	5.2	4.3	3.7	3.3	2.9	2.6
675	-	9	6.8	5.4	4.5	3.9	3.4	3	2.7
700	-	-	7	5.6	4.7	4	3.5	3.1	2.8

Step 1: Start here. Begin by finding the CALORIES of your food item from top to bottom.
Step 2: Find the GRAMS from left to right across the page here.
The number at that intersection is The Diet Denominator.

	275	300	325	350	375	400	425	450	475
50	0.2	0.2	0.2	0.1	0.1	0.1	0.1	0.1	0.1
75	0.3	0.3	0.2	0.2	0.2	0.2	0.2	0.2	0.2
100	0.4	0.3	0.3	0.3	0.3	0.3	0.2	0.2	0.2
125	0.5	0.4	0.4	0.4	0.3	0.3	0.3	0.3	0.3
150	0.5	0.5	0.5	0.4	0.4	0.4	0.4	0.3	0.3
175	0.6	0.6	0.5	0.5	0.5	0.4	0.4	0.4	0.4
200	0.7	0.7	0.6	0.6	0.5	0.5	0.5	0.4	0.4
225	0.8	0.8	0.7	0.6	0.6	0.6	0.5	0.5	0.5
250	0.9	0.8	0.8	0.7	0.7	0.6	0.6	0.6	0.5
275	1	0.9	0.8	0.8	0.7	0.7	0.6	0.6	0.6
300	1.1	1	0.9	0.9	0.8	0.8	0.7	0.7	0.6
325	1.2	1.1	1	0.9	0.9	0.8	0.8	0.7	0.7
350	1.3	1.2	1.1	1	0.9	0.9	0.8	0.8	0.7
375	1.4	1.3	1.2	1.1	1	0.9	0.9	0.8	0.8
400	1.5	1.3	1.2	1.1	1.1	1	0.9	0.9	0.8
425	1.5	1.4	1.3	1.2	1.1	1.1	1	0.9	0.9
450	1.6	1.5	1.4	1.3	1.2	1.1	1.1	1	0.9
475	1.7	1.6	1.5	1.4	1.3	1.2	1.1	1.1	1
500	1.8	1.7	1.5	1.4	1.3	1.3	1.2	1.1	1.1
525	1.9	1.8	1.6	1.5	1.4	1.3	1.2	1.2	1.1
550	2	1.8	1.7	1.6	1.5	1.4	1.3	1.2	1.2
575	2.1	1.9	1.8	1.6	1.5	1.4	1.4	1.3	1.2
600	2.2	2	1.8	1.7	1.6	1.5	1.4	1.3	1.3
625	2.3	2.1	1.9	1.8	1.7	1.6	1.5	1.4	1.3
650	2.4	2.2	2	1.9	1.7	1.6	1.5	1.4	1.4
675	2.5	2.3	2.1	1.9	1.8	1.7	1.6	1.5	1.4
700	2.5	2.3	2.2	2	1.9	1.8	1.6	1.6	1.5

For this plan to be successful, it is helpful, but not necessary for you to understand in greater detail how this plan works. It is especially helpful if you are able to provide examples of how this plan works that make common sense to your individual lifestyle. Lastly, it is essential that you are able to begin to select food items based on this plan. Now you are prepared to use this plan as a part of your daily routine and you can truly begin to benefit.

The average Diet Denominator of homemade food items is about 3; however, energy dense foods such as many common foods from the grocery store commonly fall between 4 and sometimes as high as 6 or even higher on *The Diet Denominator* scale. As you now know, the variety in *The Diet Denominator* scale among various food items is possible because in addition to fats, carbohydrates, and/or proteins, most foods contain some proportion of water and fiber. Let's look at some examples illustrated in the table below.

Table 6   *The Diet Denominator* of Some High Energy Density Foods

Food Item	Food Energy (calories)	Weight (grams)	Diet Denominator
Pecans, halves	720	108	6.7
Brazil nuts	185	28	6.5
Walnuts, English, pieces	180	28	6.3
Mixed nuts with peanuts, oil, salted	175	28	6.2
Pork, cured, bacon, regular	110	19	5.8
Corn chips	155	28	5.5
Milk chocolate candy, with almonds	150	28	5.3
Potato chips	105	20	5.3
Noodles, chow mein, canned	220	45	4.9
Salami, dry type	85	20	4.3
Doughnuts, cake type, plain	210	50	4.2
Onion rings, breaded, frozen, prepared	80	20	4.0

http://www.nal.usda.gov/fnic/foodcomp/Data/

As you will learn, choosing food items with a Diet Denominator at or around 3 or below is a great place to start with this diet because that is the average Diet Denominator of many common home-made foods. And if you are like most of us, the average Diet Denominator of most of what you eat is higher than that.

This can be explained by the fact that *The Diet Denominator* of foods can vary widely, that means that there are lots of foods with a good Diet Denominator left to choose from while there are plenty that you can avoid which are otherwise parts of your normal diet. If you eat most foods at or below the average energy content (energy lean food choices) the result will be that you consume fewer calories.

In comparison to the table illustrating food items with a high Diet Denominator, Table 7 illustrates more common food items some with a high and some with a low Diet Denominator. Taken together, a comparison of these tables illustrates the fact that there is enough variability in *The Diet Denominator* of foods to allow you to select less energy dense food items while still choosing foods that you enjoy.

Let's try an example. Take a look at Table 7 below and try to calculate *The Diet Denominator* for one of the food items such as potato chips or canned tuna illustrated below.

Calculate The Diet Denominator: potato chips

105 calories / 20 grams = 5.3 on The Diet Denominator scale.

Calculate The Diet Denominator: canned tuna

135 calories / 85 grams = 1.6 on The Diet Denominator scale.

Table 7 Diet Denominator of Some Common Food Items

Description of Food	Food Energy (calories)	Weight (grams)	Diet Denominator
Mixed nuts w/ peanuts, oil, salted	175	28	6.2
Milk chocolate candy with peanuts	155	28	5.5
Potato chips	105	20	5.3
Noodles, chow mein, canned	220	45	4.9
Nature valley granola cereal	125	28	4.4
Pork chop, loin, panfry, lean	335	89	3.8
Wheat cereal	100	28	3.5
Frankfurter, cooked	145	45	3.2
Ground beef, broiled, lean	230	85	2.7
Veal rib, med fat, roasted	230	85	2.7
Taco	195	81	2.4
Pancakes, plain, homemade	60	27	2.2
Turkey, roasted, dark meat	160	85	1.9
Avocados, California	305	173	1.8
Tuna, canned, drained, water, white	135	85	1.6
Turkey, roasted, light meat	135	85	1.6
Flounder or sole, baked, margarine	120	85	1.4
Spaghetti, meatballs, tomato sauce, canned	260	250	1.0
Apricots, dried, cooked, unsweetened	210	250	0.8
Peaches, raw, sliced	75	170	0.4
Broccoli, raw, cooked, drained	45	155	0.3
Peppers, sweet, raw, green	20	74	0.3

http://www.nal.usda.gov/fnic/foodcomp/Data/

For a more complete table of some common foods, look in Appendix 3. With this plan, you are avoiding the foods that are energy dense while choosing foods that are energy lean thereby eating fewer calories. As a quick exercise, review the tables above and see how many calories you could save by selecting energy lean items you enjoy over energy dense items you would otherwise have selected. Feel free to use other tables in this book or calculate The Diet Denominator for other food items to do this exercise.

The important thing is that you learn how much you could benefit from this plan. As you learn more about this plan you will realize that foods such as soups and stews make great food choices based on *The Diet Denominator* and based on their energy density. However, most choices are not that obvious.

While *The Diet Denominator* is based on the energy density of foods, this plan does not restrict you to complex charts or pyramids, expensive menus, or commit to memory what foods you can choose. Additionally, utilization of the plan is not restricted to your home. This plan demonstrates how to easily pick the best foods for your weight-loss goals complete with real-world examples of foods you are already familiar with from fast food restaurants. *The Diet Denominator* takes this concept one significant step further in that it provides a way to apply the plan to your everyday life. As a result, *The Diet Denominator* demonstrates in simple terms how you can easily change your eating habits and make educated food choices in an effort to lose weight more easily and effectively.

There is no easier formula, theory, or method that assists you in evaluating which foods you should select in a store, restaurant, or at home than this plan. This plan allows you to select the right food choices easily and without limiting your food choices drastically like most other plans. Perhaps even more importantly, you do not need purchase expensive premade meals, understand complex pyramids, or to shop in only one row of the grocery store.

You will be surprised at what foods have a high and a low Diet Denominator and at how easy cutting calories without reducing the volume of food you consume can become all without feeling hungry as with other plans. With this plan, you are avoiding the foods that are energy dense while choosing foods that are energy lean. As a quick exercise, review the tables above and see how many calories you could save by selecting energy lean items you enjoy over energy dense items you would otherwise have selected.

*Did you know? You can use **ounces** instead of grams to calculate The Diet Denominator. If you absolutely wish to avoid using grams, simply divide the calories per serving by the ounces per serving. As such, foods with a Diet Denominator of 56 to 85 are comparable to foods with a Diet Denominator of 2 to 3 using grams and make better (energy lean) choices while foods with a Diet Denominator of 140 to 168 are comparable to foods with a Diet Denominator of 5 to 6 and make less optimal (energy dense) choices. The total scale for ounces is from 0 to 250 instead of 0 to 9. Another way to put it, multiply The Diet Denominator using grams by 28 to get The Diet Denominator using ounces or divide The Diet Denominator using ounces by 0.035 to get The Diet Denominator using grams.*

In conclusion, *The Diet Denominator* consists of a diet plan complete with a food evaluation tool for use in your everyday life allowing you to evaluate homemade foods, fast foods, and grocery food items so that you can make informed food choices and lose weight incrementally over time. To lose weight, simply select more items with a Diet Denominator at or below average food items (around 3), or calculate your magic number, which is a way to personalize this diet plan to each individual and will be discussed in the coming chapters.

Take home messages

- *The Diet Denominator* consists of a diet plan complete with a food evaluation tool for use as part of your daily routine
- *The Diet Denominator* is simple and easy to use. There is no need to memorize which food items are high or low in energy density, high or low protein, good carbohydrates or bad
- The average Diet Denominator of home-cooked foods is variable, but around 3
- This number is much higher for restaurants and fast foods, and certain snack items, which is why this plan is so useful
- Choosing food items with a Diet Denominator at or around 3 or below is a great place to start with this diet because that is the average of many common home-made foods

Want to learn more? Some seemingly healthy food items that you might feel are great for dieting such as a granola bar actually have quite a bit of calories evident by their Diet Denominator. Granola, on average, has a Diet Denominator of 4.0 (less optimal choice). Meanwhile, nuts such as pecans, Brazilian nuts, and mixed nuts have a Diet Denominator of around 4-5 or more.

6. Satiety (Feeling of Fullness)

Americans and people from other industrialized nations have become accustomed to being served massive portion sizes at restaurants, fast food places, and as a result, increasingly at home. In fact, you may have noticed that serving sizes have increased steadily over the past few decades; however, hunger has not changed. Clearly, we don't walk around feeling full all the time thanks to the increased serving sizes, wouldn't you agree?

The feeling of fullness is termed satiety. Satiety is that feeling you get after you eat a satisfying meal, and it has gained increasing attention particularly among researchers in recent years. For example, research has shown that certain foods have a greater effect on the feeling of fullness. In fact, certain foods make us feel full more than others. You might be surprised as to what foods makes you feel full, and more surprised at what foods you probably eat on a regular basis that don't make you feel full. Just to put this into perspective, Table 8 demonstrates the serving sizes of a few common food items today compared with 20 years ago. You will notice that not only has the serving size and number of calories increased, but the energy density of these items has increased as well. This indicates that a simple portion control diet will not work.

For example, a simple cup of coffee has doubled in size (a factor of 2) from 8 **fluid ounces** just 20 years ago to 16 fluid ounces today. Perhaps more importantly, this doubling in size came with an increase from 45 calories to 350 calories (a factor of nearly 8) not just because there is twice as much coffee, but largely because the various condiments and items added to the coffee. Therefore, the importance of *The Diet Denominator* in choosing food items as they are labeled today can't be overstated.

Table 8   Changes in Food Portion Sizes in Recent Years[12]

	20 years ago		Today	
Food Item	**Serving Size**	**Calories**	**Serving Size**	**Calories**
Coffee	8 oz	45	16	350
Blueberry Muffin	1.5 oz	210	5 oz	500
Pepperoni pizza	2 slices	500	2 slices	850

Even when served in ample serving sizes, foods that have a high energy density and thus are high in calories do not necessarily increase satiety or make you feel full. Interestingly, most people are surprised when they learn that foods that have a greater energy density, such as fatty foods, do not necessarily make them feel full. Perhaps more importantly, you are more likely to eat more later on in the day after eating these types of foods adding to your daily caloric intake. This is important because eating foods that do not help to make you feel full, result in you eating more food and consuming more calories either between meals or at the next meal resulting in weight gain over time. This can make dieting an uphill struggle. Thus, there is no real benefit to eating foods that do not make you feel full and perhaps more importantly, such foods are generally of poor nutritional value.

Did you know? Processed foods often lose valuable nutrients. During processing, some of these nutrients are added back; however, many believe that the whole is greater than the sum of the parts. In other words, simply adding select nutrients back does not necessarily have the same properties.

Fullness is caused by a variety of factors, one of which is the amount (volume) of the food consumed. Unlike carbohydrates and fat, it is the protein, fiber, and water content of foods that helps make us feel full. With this diet plan, you can "you're your tank for less" by consuming an equal or larger portion of food while consuming fewer calories.

Let's look at an example. We have all eaten countless potatoes in our lifetimes and will likely continue to eat many more. As illustrated in Figure 11, you can eat a significantly greater portion size of mashed potatoes compared with French fried potatoes. This is because the energy density if far greater in French fries. For

---

[12] For more information, visit the Department of Health and Humans Services website available at: http://hp2010.nhlbihin.net/portion/

example, Wendy's medium French fries have 430 calories per 142 grams, for a Diet Denominator of 3.0. A Wendy's baked potato with butter has 320 calories per 294 grams, a Diet Denominator of 1.1. Choosing the baked potato offers nearly twice as much food by weight yet contains nearly 25% less calories. Thus, the volume of food you can eat to consume the same or fewer calories are far greater for the baked potato, making you feel fuller, longer.

Figure 11 Fried versus baked potatoes

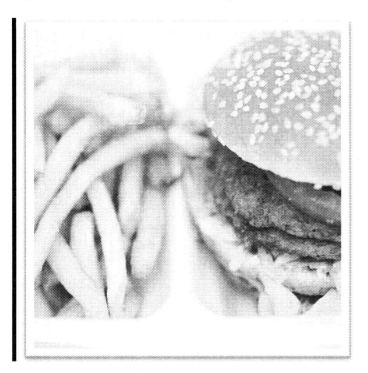

Each time you make a choice based on *The Diet Denominator*, you begin consuming less energy dense food items while feeling more satisfied. If you continue to make such choices, these differences will add up over time helping you achieve your weight loss goals. You should be beginning to see how simply decreasing the portion size of the foods that you eat is not the answer to a successful diet. Eating less French fries is not going to help you lose weight? Think about it. Simply consuming less of a poor diet that is high in calories, low in nutrients, and not very satisfying, or filling is not likely to be sustainable let alone successful or healthy. Alternatively, a diet plan that helps you to make informed food choices and that is easy to use and understand, is much more likely to help you reach your end goal.

Use the blank table below to see how many calories you could save in a week by choosing one item with a recommended Diet Denominator over another item that you otherwise might have chosen.

Table 9   Calculate your Calorie Savings using *The Diet Denominator*

Item	Calories	Grams	Diet Denominator
Old item			
New item			
Difference per sitting			
Difference per week			

In addition to eating foods with a low Diet Denominator, eating foods that increase satiety is another way to consume fewer calories while consuming a greater proportion of foods that can make you feel full. Choosing foods with a good Diet Denominator value will help you to eat an adequate volume of food while feeling full and consuming fewer calories. However, not all foods with a low Diet Denominator will make you feel full. Think of this plan as more of path in the right direction. A plan such as this is a great place to start because with this plan you will begin to consume fewer calories while feeling less hungry, begin to eat a healthier diet, and you will learn how to select the best foods on your own over time.

Water is the most abundant chemical in the body making up roughly 60% of your bodyweight. Water serves as a solvent and aids in the transport of certain chemical and nutrients throughout the body. Water also helps to eliminate toxins and waste from the body. Given these facts, it is no surprise that the water content of the foods that you eat is important. In fact, thirst can be mistaken for hunger.

One item that contributes to the volume of foods without adding calories is water. Water contributes to the volume of foods without adding to the number of calories is water. The water of content of foods varies widely. Foods with high water content help us to consume fewer calories.

Table 10 contains information on the water content of some high water content and low water content foods for comparison. Choosing foods with higher water content can lead to the consumption of fewer calories while feeling less hungry. Ultimately, you could consume up to three times the high water content foods while eating consuming less calories than low water content foods.

Table 10   Water Content of Some High and Low Water Content Foods

Food Item	Water Content (%)
High Water Content	
Cucumbers Raw	96%
Lettuce Head	96%
Squash Boiled	96%
Radishes Raw	95%
Celery	94%
Low Water Content	
Coconut Dried	7%
Pecans	7%
Walnuts	4%
Peanuts Shelled	Trace
Peanut Butter	Trace

The water content of food has the biggest effect on the energy density. In an article appearing in the American Journal of Clinical Nutrition in 2007, it was concluded that after a year-long clinical trial in obese women, consuming energy lean food items such as fruits and vegetables compared with a low fat diet resulted in participants reporting decreased feelings of hunger. [13]

---

[13] Ello-Martin JA. *Am J Clin Nutr.* 2007 Jun;85(6):1465-77.

Table 11 Fiber Content of Some High and Low Fiber Content Foods

Food Item	Fiber Content (grams)
High Fiber Content	
Navy beans, cooked	9.5 grams per ½ cup
Whole wheat English muffin	4.4 grams per muffin
Brown Rice, uncooked	5.5 grams per ½ cup
Whole Grains (wheat, oats, barley)	Variable
Lima beans, cooked	6.6 grams per ½ cup
Low Fiber Foods	
Meats (steak, hamburger, pork chops, and turkey)	Trace
Seafood (Clams, flounder, scallops, and shrimp)	Trace
Cheeses (cottage, mozzarella, and ricotta)	Trace

In addition to water, increased amounts of fiber in a food item can help make you feel less hungry while consuming fewer calories (Table 11). Thus, most foods with a low Diet Denominator have high fiber or water content (increased volume), which can add to the volume of food you consume helping you to feel full. Fiber increases satiety in another way. Fiber increases digestion time meaning that foods high in fiber take longer for your body to digest thereby making you feel more satisfied for longer and decreasing hunger. Fiber also traps some fat in your intestines so that you do not absorb the calories in some foods. Clearly, foods with high water and/or fiber content help to explain how volumetric (energy density) diet plans work to help you to feel full and eat less.

High-fiber foods make an excellent choice. High fiber snacks include popcorn, oriental mix (rice based), whole wheat pretzels, granola bar (fruit filled), sun chips, and rice cakes (brown rice). Other high fiber items include rye wafers, cornbread, rye bread, bran muffins, and whole wheat dinner rolls. In addition to fiber and the volume of food that you eat, the protein in food helps to make you feel full particularly when compared with the calories in the food. Choosing foods with a good Diet Denominator value can increase you feeling of fullness. Eating foods that increase your feeling of fullness will result in your consuming fewer calories over time because you get full sooner and eat less afterwards, which is the key to losing weight and maintaining your weight loss.

In fact, while the evidence is conflicting, on a calorie to calorie basis, a great deal of research indicates that protein has the greatest effect on satiety thus protein has the greatest influence on feeling full. [14,15]

Lastly, liquids can be compared using *The Diet Denominator*. To do so, it is assumed that 1 gram is equal to 1 mL of liquid, which is pretty accurate given most food and drink items. This is possible because of the fact that the density (mass in grams/volume in mL) of water is 1.0, which is the mass. Note: for these purposes, it is safe to compare 1 mL of liquid of food to 1 gram of food.

Diet Denominator Facts: If you are trying to **gain** weight, you will want to be sure to avoid eating the soup at your favorite lunch-buffet. However, it you wish to **reduce your calorie intake** by 100-200 calories a day, eat foods such as soup, stew, and fruits with a high water content before your meal. You may have heard that drinking water before a meal reduces hunger. Unfortunately, the effect is short lived. However, in a study at Pennsylvania State University, researchers compared the effects of drinking water with a pre-meal, to consuming a soup pre-meal made with the same ingredients on hunger and satiety. When the participants consumed the chunky-soup, their caloric intake at lunch was reduced by 13-16%, suggesting that water incorporated into a meal decreases hunger and energy intake throughout the day. This likely occurs because the watered-down food has a lower energy density (calories per gram) much like carbohydrates and proteins have fewer calories per gram than fat and nutritive liquids stay in the stomach longer leading to fullness, which over the course of a year could add up to thousands.[16]

---

[14] Barkeling B, Rössner S, Björvell H. Effects of a high-protein meal (meat) and a high-carbohydrate meal (vegetarian) on satiety measured by automated computerized monitoring of subsequent food intake, motivation to eat and food preferences. *Int J Obes.* 1990;14(9):743-51.

[15] Stubbs RJ. Macronutrient effects on appetite. *Int J Obes Relat Metab Disord.* 1995;19 Suppl 5:S11-9.

[16] Rolls B et al. Water incorporated into a food but not served with a food decreases energy intake in lean women. *Am J Clin Nutr.* 1999. 70(4):448-55.

In conclusion, choosing foods that increase satiety can result in your eating a similar volume of food while consuming fewer calories compared with consuming an equal volume of more energy dense food. That is to say, you can eat foods that are energy lean without having to feel hungry while remaining on your diet and you will not be as hungry between meals. With *The Diet Denominator*, you can eat foods that are energy lean and get the same feeling of fullness. The key is to know which foods to choose. In fact, with *The Diet Denominator*, you will learn to choose foods that are energy lean and that increase your feeling of fullness. Energy lean foods are generally healthier, because energy dense foods are often high fat and low in essential micronutrients thus of lower quality.

Did you know? In a review article by Douglas Paddon-Jones et al, it was stated that obesity is a major health concern and that to be successful, treatment interventions must be personalized while limiting energy intake. One way to do this is to moderately increase protein intake. As a result, this could increase satiety, increase **thermogenesis** *(your body's burning of energy naturally), and help to increase or maintain fat-free muscle mass, which has various beneficial effects on the body such as improving its metabolic profile, such as by improving the ratio of good to bad cholesterol, and by lowering the overall concentration of lipids in the blood.* [17]

---

[17] Paddon-Jones D. *Am J Clin Nutr*. 2008 May;87(5):1558S-1561S. Protein, weight management, and satiety.

Take home messages

- On a calorie-for-calorie basis, protein has the greatest effect on satiety thus protein has the greatest influence on feeling full
- Thirst can often be mistaken as hunger, leading us to eat more; therefore, it is important to remain hydrated. Eating foods that contain water is helpful
- The volume of food also has a big effect on feeling full, which is mostly influenced by water content
- Foods that have a large volume but are low in calories such as soup and stew have a good Diet Denominator value and are filling due to the high water content and thus volume of food
- Portion control is often not an adequate diet plan because it leaves you feeling full
- The number of calories in a food item contributes very little to its ability to make you feel full
- Water does not contain food calories; however, the amount of water in a food items contributes benificially to the calories per gram of a food item
- In addition to water content, the fiber content of foods contributes significantly to the energy density of foods and fiber can help to reduced the absorption of fat

---

Want to learn more? Have you ever wondered why you are able to consume so much at an all you can eat buffet compared to a normal meal? Well, there is something to be said about variety, particularly when it comes to your diet. A diet full of variety in terms of food choices leads to increased consumption and greater weight gain. This is due to satiety in that diets with greater variety are less likely to make you feel full compared with a diet with less variety. Decreased variety within a meal helps to increase satiety. The benefits of eating a diet with less variety are evident in a paper by Raynor et al (2004). [18] In this study of overweight men and women, over 200 participants were randomly assigned to one of two diet routines that consisted of exercise and other behavioral treatments and the same diet. Those who consumed a diet with a decreased variety in high-fat foods and fats, oils and sweets were associated with reduced percent dietary fat consumed and weight loss. Therefore, variety in a diet plan (such as with *The Diet Denominator*) might help adopting and maintaining a low fat and low energy density diet and weight loss.

---

[18] Raynor HA et al. Relationship between changes in food group variety, dietary intake, and weight during obesity treatment. *Int J Obes*. 2004;28, 813–820.

7. Fill Your Tank for Less

In the last chapter you learned about the concept of satiety (feeling of fullness) and that some foods make you feel more satisfied than others and that the caloric content of foods has little to do with making you feel full. So naturally, it is only appropriate that there is an entire chapter dedicated to explaining the meaning of this important concept. So what is meant by the phrase "fill your tank for less"? This is a simple, yet powerful message that illustrates the importance of food selection and how some foods actually make you feel full while allowing you to consuming fewer calories.

"Fill your tank for less", is a simple concept that immortalizes one of the key principles of this book. The ability to make you feel more satisfied more easily by eating less energy dense foods is possible for two reasons. With this plan you will learn how to select food items that are energy lean; therefore, you are filling up on fewer calories. In addition, this plan allows you to select food items that increase satiety (feeling of fullness), thus making you feel full. In other words, when you select foods using this plan, you will automatically be selecting foods that are energy lean and often make you feel full. As a result, you are less hungry afterwards; therefore, you will generally consume fewer calories throughout the day.

By now, we all should know and understand that deep fried, high fat, foods have a high energy density. However, for most of the food choices we make, the distinctions are far less obvious, which is where this book is especially useful.

Over time, choosing foods that are generally more energy lean will result in you consuming fewer calories particularly when those foods make you feel fuller than those high energy density foods that leave you feeling hungry. Energy lean foods have fewer calories per gram so you can eat the same volume of food while consuming fewer calories. With this plan, you can easily select food items that contain fewer calories but that also make you feel full so that you are less likely to feel the urge to snack later. Most diet plans help you to lose weight fast only to gain the weight back once you stop dieting. This plan teaches you how to select the right foods, time and time again, and is a plan for life. This way, you lose weight incrementally over time and you can continue to take the weight off while learning to select and begin to eat more nutrient dense foods over time.

We have all eaten meals that left us feeling stuffed only to feel hungry an hour later and other foods that made us feel satisfied for many hours. You learned that this is primarily due to satiety, which is closely linked to the energy density of foods. Thus, choosing energy lean foods can help you to lose weight safely and effectively over time. *The Diet Denominator* doesn't necessarily determine if a food item will make you feel full. However, foods that are high in protein, fiber, and water, as you learned, have properties that tend to make you feel full and these foods generally have a good Diet Denominator so these concepts are closely related.

Surely you can guess some of the better food choices on a menu (French fries vs. baked potatoes, for example); however, this plan helps you to make good selections that are not so obvious and avoid other foods that you might have thought to be better (energy lean) choices. Best of all, you likely already eat and enjoy many of these foods, but with this plan you will select these and other energy lean foods while avoiding energy dense foods. Because this plan helps you make informed food choices, you still get to select the foods you want, so long as they are energy lean, which will leave you feeling more satisfied.

Food comes with a cost in terms of the number of calories per day that we consume. The effects of eating too many calories can lead to unwanted weight gain. As a result, eating too many calories becomes increasingly important as we age, because we need fewer calories to maintain our bodyweight plus we are less active and often eating more food. Therefore, for any diet plan to be successful, you have to stick with it for a prolonged period of time. Eating too many calories is important particularly as you get older because the average American gains about 10 pounds per decade of life after about 30 years of age. This is especially difficult to prevent when we eat foods high in calories that are not filling. Despite this fact, most of us eat the same if not more food, and thus calories, as we get older. With *The Diet Denominator*, you will learn that you can "fill your tank for less". That is to say, you can get full while consuming fewer calories simply by selecting foods that are energy lean while eating the same volume of food. What's more, this is not just in terms of the cost in calories but the toll that eating high energy foods, which are often of lower quality, have on your body.

> *Diet Denominator Facts:* There are 3500 calories per pound of fat weight loss. In other words, if you eat just 100 calories a day more than you burn through exercise, daily activities, and your body's normal metabolic activities, you would gain approximately 1 pound per month.

Here is an example as to how filling your tank for less can save you calories leading to weight loss over time. If you consume a 2500 calorie per day diet, you can eat 714 grams of food with an average Diet Denominator of 3.5 or 1000 grams (30% more) with an average Diet Denominator of 2.5. This reduction can lead to weight reduction over time. Here is a specific example of how you can use this plan to reduce your caloric intake with just one food item. An ordinary slice of American cheese has 60 calories per 19 grams of which 45 calories are from fat and has a Diet Denominator of 3.1. Compare that with a slice of American-style soy cheese, which has 40 calories per 17 grams with only 25 calories from fat and a Diet Denominator of just 2.3. That is a simple way to save 20 calories, all from fat while only eating 3 grams less food, which you would not even notice.

With *The Diet Denominator*, the greater the shift in the energy density of the food items you are accustomed to eating to what you choose to eat with this plan the faster and more weight you can lose without feeling hungry. Here are some examples of some simple ways to fill your tank for less.

Did you know? Soft tofu makes a great addition to your repertoire of good meals. It absorbs the flavor of whatever you cook it with and it comes as a large cube in water and is easy to prepare. It is often cut up into smaller cubes for cooking while the remainder can be stored in water for several days once opened (see instructions on the label). A standard serving contains about 60 calories and 80 grams for a Diet Denominator below 1.0. A single serving has 6 grams of soy protein and about 3 grams of fat. This makes a great replacement for chicken or beef and works great with The Diet Denominator, in part, because of its high water content.

Calculate The Diet Denominator: tofu

60 calories / 80 grams = 0.75 on The Diet Denominator scale

Fill your tank for less: Beef, chicken or tofu

Sirloin beef tips trimmed to low fat has 371 calories per 261 grams for a Diet Denominator of 1.4.

Calculate The Diet Denominator: sirloin beef

371 calories / 261 grams = 1.4 on The Diet Denominator scale

In comparison, a very healthy option such as skinless chicken breast meat which contains 78 calories per 71 grams has a Diet Denominator of 1.1.

Calculate The Diet Denominator: skinless chicken breast

78 calories / 71 grams = 1.1 on The Diet Denominator scale

Meanwhile, tofu contains about 60 calories per 80 grams for a Diet Denominator of 0.75, by far the best option.

Calculate The Diet Denominator: tofu

60 calories / 80 grams = 0.75 on The Diet Denominator scale

Did you know? That the fortune cookie you eat after a chinese dinner adds an additional 30 calories in just 8 grams for a Diet Denominator of ~3.5, while you may want to avoid the calories, it never hurts to read the fortune!

Calculate The Diet Denominator: fortune cookie

30 calories / 8 grams = 3.5 on The Diet Denominator scale

Take home messages

- With *The Diet Denominator* you can "fill your tank for less" meaning you can consume the same volume of food while consuming fewer calories by consuming energy lean foods or you can consume foods that tend to make you feel full, and these foods are often one and the same
- The volume of the food you consume, the protein, and fiber content of foods all contribute to the feeling of fullness; whereas, the fat content of foods have little effect on the feeling of fullness
- This plan allows you to select food items that increase satiety (feeling of fullness), thus making you feel full
- When you "fill your tank for less", you can consume fewer calories incrementally over time resulting in weight loss that you can keep off and result in lifestyle changes
- Generally speaking, foods with a lower energy density are healthier, so you will be eating a healthier diet when using this plan

Want to learn more? Your resting metabolic rate (RMR) is the amount of energy that your body burns while you are at rest while your body is actively performing various metabolic processes such as digestion, tissue repair, keeping you warm, breathing to name a few things. You can increase your RMR by working out and building muscle because muscles burn energy even while resting. Here is an example. Let us say that, for example, your current diet is costing you, 3000 calories/day. This leads to the accumulation of bodyweight in the form of fat year after year. However, with *The Diet Denominator* let's say you only consume 2500 calories/day while consuming the same volume of food without feeling hungry. By avoiding those 500 calories per day, you could lose over 4 pounds in just one month.

8. What is your magic number?

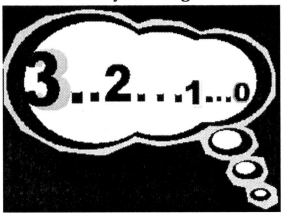

One of the best things about this plan is that it is not overly restrictive or impossible to follow. While other plans are so generalized that you are left with few food options or forced to choose from the same items over and over, this plan allows you to choose from any food items you wish, so long as you choose items that are energy lean. But as you will learn, with this plan, you can use what you have learned about *The Diet Denominator* and take it one step further by customizing the plan to your individual needs. Another advantage of this diet plan is that it can easily be customized to your specific needs. We are all different in terms of our dieting preferences, dieting needs, and dieting goals.

The concept "So what is your magic number", the focus of this chapter, allows you to customize this diet plan based on your dieting goals and prior eating habits, both of which differ for us all. Here is how it works. Start by determining your magic number, which is the average Diet Denominator of your ordinary diet then begin selecting food items at or below that number. Therefore, even those with poor eating habits can improve their diets incrementally with this plan. It's that simple.

Remember, to calculate *The Diet Denominator* for any given food item, take the calories and divide that number by the grams each from one serving, which equals *The Diet Denominator*.

Calculate The Diet Denominator: refried beans, canned

217 calories / 238 grams = 0.9 on The Diet Denominator scale

If you add up *The Diet Denominator* of say 10 of the most common food items from your normal diet and divide that number by 10 (or the number of items you wish to average), that number equals your magic number.

Use Table 12 to calculate your magic number. The try choosing foods at or below your magic number and you will begin consuming fewer calories.

Table 12   Calculate your Magic Number

Item	Calories	Grams	Diet Denominator
Example: refried beans, canned	*217*	*238*	*0.9*
1.			
2.			
3.			
4.			
5.			
6.			
7.			
8.			
9.			
10.			
Total	**Sum =**	**Sum =**	**Average =**
Diet Denominator = calories/grams Average Diet Denominator = sum of calories / sum of grams above			

As a result, you can consume fewer calories over time at your own pace based on your previous dieting habits. Therefore, with *The Diet Denominator*, you can customize your diet by calculate your magic number. Instead of choosing foods with the recommended Diet Denominator of around 3.0 or below, take the average Diet Denominator of the most common food items in your previous diet, and calculate your magic number. Thus, your magic number is unique, and equals *The Diet Denominator* of ordinary food items in your previous diet. Your magic number might be 3.0, 3.5, or even higher depending on your prior eating habits.

With *The Diet Denominator*, you simply need to select food items with a Diet Denominator at or below your magic number to begin making smart and informed food choices that will result in consuming fewer calories and losing weight incrementally over time.

With your magic number, simply begin choosing foods with a Diet Denominator at or below your magic number to begin losing weight safely and effectively. If the food item is below your magic number, it is a better (energy lean) choice.

If you want to increase your ability to lose weight over time, lower your magic number so that you can make greater gains. You can move your magic number based on how serious you are with your diet. If you want to lose more weight or lose weight faster, lower your magic number. Want to take a break from the diet plan, raise your number a bit. Utilizing your magic number will allow you to regulate how fast and how much weight you can lose and how strict of a diet you will need to consume. Best of all, this enables you to individualize your diet.

If you are preparing to use this plan but you previously had a less optimal (energy dense) diet, you can adjust your diet incrementally using *The Diet Denominator* and improve your diet incrementally over time. This prevents the "shock and awe" diet, which most people simply end up quitting.

Customization is important for long-term weight loss. It is not reasonable or realistic for someone who is overweight or particularly someone who is obese to eat a single premade, 12 ounce meal for breakfast, lunch and dinner or to eat a low calorie diet for an extended period of time even though weight loss is sure to result. Unfortunately, hunger is a powerful force and a highly restrictive diet is not feasible in these situations. Once you are aware of how to choose foods with this tool you will be eating a healthier diet and eating foods with a higher nutritional value. This is beneficial for your overall health because energy dense foods are generally of poor quality because high fat foods contain less of the important micronutrients and more empty calories.

> *Did you know? According to the U.S. Department of Agriculture (USDA) Dietary Guidelines for Americans, 2005 (www.healthierus.gov/dietaryguidelines), "Many Americans consume more calories than they need without meeting recommended intakes for a number of nutrients. This circumstance means that most people need to choose meals and snacks that are high in nutrients but low to moderate in energy content; that is, meeting nutrient recommendations must go hand in hand with keeping calories under control. Doing so offers important benefits—normal growth and development of children, health promotion for people of all ages, and reduction of risk for a number of chronic diseases that are major public health problems."*

Even those with poor eating habits can improve their diets incrementally by using this plan. Simply calculate *The Diet Denominator* for any food item at home, in the grocery store, even fast foods. If *The Diet Denominator* is below around 3.0 it's a better (energy lean) choice.

Interestingly, *The Diet Denominator* works with liquid foods like soup and can be used to compare liquids to one another such as various juices, sodas, and other beverages. This is possible because it can be assumed that 1 mL of liquid equals about 1 gram of food. Therefore, *The Diet Denominator* for liquid foods or beverages is the number of calories per serving divided by the number of mL's instead of grams. Finally, with your magic number, if you are not experiencing the results you want, simply start to incrementally decrease your magic number.

Using the blank table below, record some of your favorite foods with a Diet Denominator at or below your magic number so that you can choose these foods in the future. You will find that you already enjoyed some foods with a good Diet Denominator and that you enjoy others you did not realized had a good Diet Denominator, some of which you might otherwise have forgotten you enjoy that have a good Diet Denominator if you did not make a note of them.

Plus, any types of record of your progress, serves as positive reinforcement, which helps you to succeed and provides a reason to congratulate yourself for a job well done. Use Table 13 to make a note of your favorite foods with the recommended Diet Denominator so you remember to choose them in the future. Review Appendix 4 to find more typical foods with a recommended Diet Denominator.

Table 13   Diet Denominator of your Favorite Foods

Food Item	Calories	Grams	Diet Denominator
Example: refried beans, canned	*217*	*238*	*0.9*
1.			
2.			
3.			
4.			
5.			
6.			
7.			
8.			
9.			
10.			

Take home messages

- Your magic number allows you to customize this diet plan based on your dieting goals and prior eating habits
- Your magic number is the average Diet Denominator of your ordinary diet
- To begin losing weight, simply select food items at or below your magic number
- If you are not experiencing the results you want, be sure you are sticking to your plan and if so, simply start to incrementally decrease your magic number
- *The Diet Denominator* for liquid foods or beverages is the number of calories per serving divided by the number of mL's instead of grams

Want to learn more? Trainers and exercise enthusiasts recommend a protein shake after a workout. Recent evidence suggests that after a workout your body needs to replenish the used up energy for critical processes and so that it is available again. One way the body can replace this energy is from **amino acids** from the proteins in your muscles, which can serve as a warehouse of energy when necessary. While amino acids do not serve as significant sources of energy under normal circumstances, they might provide an estimated 3-6% of the energy produced during exercise. Since you workout hard to build or at least tone your muscles, and muscles burn energy naturally, you do not want this to happen. One way to prevent or lessen this is to consume a protein bar or protein drink after a workout. This will give you body the energy it needs while sparing you muscles. Energy and other drinks contain calories, therefore be sure to fit them into a sensible diet plan. [19]

---

[19] M.J. Gibala. Regulation of skeletal muscle amino acid metabolism during exercise. *International Journal of Sports Nutrition and Exercise Metabolism.* 2001. 11(1):87-108.

9. How do snack foods measure up to *The Diet Denominator*?

If you recall, the average Diet Denominator of the ordinary food items prepared from items from the grocery store is around 3.0 and to lose weight, you want to try and choose foods with a Diet Denominator at or below this number or below your magic number. Keep in mind that this number can be much higher for fast foods and even snack foods, which is why this plan is so useful.

Comparing various snack food items using *The Diet Denominator* is fun, easy, and interesting because you won't believe some of the results. So throw away that granola bar and read about how *The Diet Denominator* even helps you to choose the best snack foods.

You might be aware that heavily flavored, buttery popcorn has more calories per serving than fat-free popcorn, but you will surely be surprised at some of the results revealed in this book. While popcorn does contain some fiber, the butter and/or seasonings often contain many of the calories thus these make a less optimal (energy dense) food choice. For example, the amount of calories in popcorn flavoring other than butter is astonishing.

Fill your tank for less: low-fat vs. cheese flavored popcorn

Low-fat microwave popcorn has 119 calories (24 from fat) per 28 grams for a Diet Denominator of 4.3, which is a less optimal choice.

Calculate The Diet Denominator: low-fat popcorn

119 calories / 28 grams = 4.3 on The Diet Denominator scale

However, cheese flavored popcorn has 148 calories (81 from fat) per 28 grams, for a Diet Denominator of 5.3.

Calculate The Diet Denominator: cheese flavored popcorn

148 calories / 28 grams = 5.3 on The Diet Denominator scale

Therefore, the original flavored popcorn makes a much better alternative. Thus, it is not always about making the best choice, but sometimes just making a better choice. While neither is an optimal choice, with this plan, you can easily make the better choice, saving you calories one handful at a time. With this example, you should be able to see how you can benefit from this plan quickly and easily. This example illustrates that you can eat the same amount of food (28 grams) while consuming 29 fewer calories and 57 fewer calories from fat by choosing the regular popcorn over the cheese flavored popcorn.

As a test, find snack foods that you might normally select and then items to replace them with using *The Diet Denominator*. Can you see the difference? In fact, some snacks that you might not have otherwise chosen make good snacks with this plan.

Did you know? Eggs make a great snack food. They can be hard boiled, in the form of egg salad, or even poached if you have the time.

In fact, a hard-boiled egg has about 75 calories per 50 grams for a Diet Denominator of 1.5. This slightly better than a whole, fried egg, which has about 90 calories per 50 grams for a Diet Denominator of 1.8.

Fill your tank for less: Chocolate instant pudding vs. potato chips

Instant pudding has 155 calories per 130 grams, for a Diet Denominator of 1.2.

Calculate The Diet Denominator: chocolate instant pudding

155 calories / 139 grams = 1.2 on The Diet Denominator scale

This makes a great (energy lean) snack. This is important because you might not have otherwise realized this was an energy lean snack, plus you are sure to enjoy it. In comparison, potato chips have 100 calories per 20 grams, which is equivalent to a Diet Denominator of 5.0, a less optimal (energy dense) choice.

Calculate The Diet Denominator: potato chips

100 calories / 20 grams = 5.0 on The Diet Denominator scale

This is a relatively easy choice. However, choosing between most snack food items is not this simple. Some of the best snack foods based on *The Diet Denominator* include cottage cheese, enchiladas, and even low-fat vanilla milkshakes! Plus, many vegetables (and fruits) which have a good Diet Denominator make great (energy lean) snack foods because they are sweet or salty to the taste making them satisfying. The facts behind which snack packs and low fat snacks make a good snack choice is also revealed using *The Diet Denominator*.

Fill your tank for less: peanut butter granola or low-fat ice cream

A peanut butter granola bar has 170 calories per 35 grams for a Diet Denominator of 4.8, and a **less optimal choice**.

Calculate The Diet Denominator: peanut butter granola bar

170 calories / 35 grams = 4.8 on The Diet Denominator scale

Whereas, a Weight Watchers™ low-fat Oreo™ Ice Cream Bar has 140 calories per 71 grams for a Diet Denominator of 2.0 making these a **better choice** thus an energy lean choice.

Calculate The Diet Denominator: Weight Watchers™ low-fat Oreo™ Ice Cream

140 calories / 71 grams = 2.0 on The Diet Denominator scale

Fill your tank for less: 100 calorie diet packs

The 100 calorie diet pack is a recent trend in the packaging and marketing of snack foods. Some are good, some not as good. But how can you tell? The answer is using *The Diet Denominator*.

For example, the Nabisco™ Oreo™ Thin 100 Calorie Pack has 100 calories per 138 grams for a Diet Denominator of 0.72, which is a **better choice**.

Calculate The Diet Denominator: Nabisco™ Oreo™ Thin 100 Calorie Pack

100 calories / 138 grams = 0.72 on The Diet Denominator scale

The Hostess™ 100 Calorie Pack Carrot Cake has 100 calories per 34 grams for a Diet Denominator of 2.9, which is a **better choice**.

Calculate The Diet Denominator: Hostess™ 100 Calorie Pack Carrot Cake

100 calories / 34 grams = 2.9 on The Diet Denominator scale

However, the Nabisco™ 100 Calorie Pack Lorna Doone™ has 100 calories per 21 grams for a Diet Denominator of 4.8, and is thus a **less optimal choice**.

Calculate The Diet Denominator: Nabisco™ 100 Calorie Pack Lorna Doone™

100 calories / 21 grams = 4.8 on The Diet Denominator scale

Table 14 below illustrates the Diet Denominator of various cookies and other snack foods.

Table 14   Diet Denominator of Various Cookies and Other Snack Foods

Description of Food	Food Energy (calories)	Weight (grams)	Diet Denominator
Sugar free flavored popsicle pops	12	55	0.2
Fast foods, nachos, with cheese, beans, ground beef, and peppers	569	255	2.2
Nachos with cheese	346	113	3.1
Animal Crackers	120	30	4.0
Archway™ Home Style Cookies, Ruth's Oatmeal	111	26	4.3
Arby™ Gourmet Chocolate Cookie	200	45	4.4
Low fat vanilla wafers	353	80	4.4
Grandma's™ Peanut Butter Cookies	370	78	4.7
Twix™, peanut butter cookie bar	311	58	5.4

Take home messages

- Some of the best tasting snacks that you might not have otherwise thought to eat make good snacks with this plan and can be eaten in place of some of the less optimal (energy dense) choices you might otherwise have consumed
- Granola and some other seemingly healthy snack foods are often high in calories and do not make good snacks with this plan
- Hidden calories are often found in snack foods such as in the flavoring in popcorn. Without the flavoring you can consume the same amount of food while consuming fewer calories
- Not only are the number of calories important, but the number of calories from fat, which you want to avoid

Want to learn more? Activia™ is a great-tasting low fat yogurt from Dannon™ that contains *Bifidus Regularis*™, a natural probiotic culture that can help regulate your digestive system by helping reduce long intestinal transit time*. *Bifidus Regularis*™, available only in Activia™, consists of a live "friendly" bacterium (singular word for bacteria) that's beneficial when eaten daily.

For more information, visit Activia™'s web site available at: www.activia.com. Interestingly, Activia™ has a Diet Denominator of 2.0.

10.   How do fast foods measure up to *The Diet Denominator*?

So you already know that fast food salads are a better choice than most other foods that are offered depending on which, and how much dressing is used to enhance the flavor or palatability of such items. In this chapter, you will be amazed at some of the food choices that represent better choices and less optimal choices based on *The Diet Denominator*. This will change the way you look at, and order, fast foods in the future.

As for restaurant foods, the larger chains list there nutritional information either on the internet or provide the information in leaflets similar to fast food restaurants on their own or due to regulatory requirements. If the calories and grams of a potential food choice is not available or easily obtainable, try using the nutrition information from the same food item available from another restaurant or grocery store, which you can find using a resource such as www.nutritiondata.com. Alternatively, draw from the information and examples in this book or use your previous experiences with this plan to make your best judgment in the rare instance when the calories and grams are not available.

Now let's take a look at some of the more common fast food items. Some of the choices are obvious, but some are not so obvious. For example, McDonalds™ Premium Grilled Chicken Classic Sandwich is 1.9; whereas, the Chicken McNuggets™ are a 3.9 and the fries are a 3.3.

Here are some more examples. KFC™'s mashed potatoes with gravy have 140 calories per 151 grams, which equals a Diet Denominator of 0.92, and makes for a better snack. Jersey Mike's™ #7 Turkey Breast submarine sandwich has 210 calories per 233 grams, which equals a Diet Denominator of 0.90, a makes for a great (energy lean) meal.

As for breakfast, these choices can be a little more difficult. Scrambled eggs come in at 1.8, while the sausage biscuit is 3.7. Quaker Instant Oatmeal (Cinnamon & Spice) breakfast has 170 calories per 46 grams plus 240 mL (grams) water, which equals a Diet Denominator of 0.6 (with water). Simply put, no plan is easier, more informative, fun or rewarding as this plan.

Diet Denominator Facts: Seltzer water is nothing more than carbonated water. It has zero calories and when served ice cold, is very refreshing. You can add zero calorie flavors to plain water or seltzer water, for a zero calorie replacement for soda.

It is important to note that *The Diet Denominator* of food items, on average, is much higher for restaurants and fast foods, which is why this plan is so useful, because you can save yourself a lot of calories by using this plan in these circumstances. To lose weight, simply choose foods with a Diet Denominator at or below the average food item. Alternatively, calculate your magic number, and select foods at or below that number to lose weight safely and effectively.

Here are some examples using some favorite fast foods. Surely you can guess some of the better choices on a menu; however, this plan helps you to choose food items that are not so obvious. The plan helps you to choose foods that are less energy dense, leaving you feeling full and consuming fewer calories.

Let's look at some examples. McDonalds™ Premium Grilled Chicken Classic Sandwich has 420 calories per 226 grams, which equals a Diet Denominator of 1.9 **(better choice)**; McDonalds™ Chicken McNuggets™ has 420 calories per 160 grams, which equals a Diet Denominator of 3.9 **(less optimal choice)**; McDonalds™ French fries has 380 calories per 114 grams, which equals a Diet Denominator of 3.3 **(less optimal choice)**; McDonalds™ scrambled eggs has 170 calories per 96 grams, which equals a Diet Denominator of 1.8 **(less optimal choice)**; McDonalds™ Sausage biscuit has 410 calories per 113 grams, which equals a Diet Denominator of 3.6 **(less optimal choice)**; Pappa John's™ The Works pizza has 330 calories per 157 grams, which equals a Diet Denominator of 2.1 **(better choice)**.

KFC™'s mashed potatoes and gravy has 140 calories per 151 grams, which equals a Diet Denominator of 0.92 **(better snack)**. Jersey Mike's™ #7 Turkey Breast submarine sandwich has 210 calories per 233 grams, which equals a Diet Denominator of 0.90 **(better choice)**.

Table 15   Common Fast Foods with a Diet Denominator below 2.5

Description of Food	Food Energy (calories)	Weight (grams)	Diet Denominator
KFC™			
Chicken breast no skin or breading	140	108	1.30
Roasted Twister without sauce	330	247	1.34
Chicken pot pie	770	423	1.82
Crispy Strips	350	151	2.32
McDonalds™			
Premium Grilled Chicken Classic Sandwich	420	226	1.86
Honey Mustard Snack Wrap™ with Grilled Chicken	260	124	2.10
Premium Grilled Chicken Ranch BLT Sandwich	520	246	2.11
Big N' Tasty™	460	206	2.23
Panda Express™			
Hot and sour soup	110	336	0.33
Beef and broccoli	150	154	0.97
Mandarin chicken	250	154	1.62
Steamed rice	380	224	1.70
Papa John's™			
Garden Fresh Pizza slice, original crust	190	104	1.83
The works slice, original crust	330	157	2.10
Cheese pizza slice, original crust	300	132	2.27
Tuscan Six Cheese, original crust	210	89	2.36
Taco Bell™			
Crunchy taco	92	150	0.61
Soft taco beef	113	180	0.63
7-layer burrito	248	380	0.65
Fiesta Taco Salad no Shell	490	479	1.02

KFC™, McDonalds™, Panda Express™, Papa John's™, and Taco Bell™ are registered trademarks of their respective parent companies.

Let's compare two seemingly similar food choices from a fast food restaurant. In Figure 12 are two a food labels both from items from a favorite fast food restaurant Taco Bell™. On the left is a food label for a bean burrito; whereas, the one on the right is for nachos. Can you guess which one has a better Diet Denominator and thus makes a better choice? You will note that the bean burrito has a Diet Denominator of 2.0; whereas, the nachos have a Diet Denominator of 3.7. At first glance, you might notice that the burrito has 42 more calories; however, it is important to note that you are also getting twice the amount of food. Thus, you would have to eat two orders of nachos to eat the same amount (in grams) of food as in the burrito and that would give you nearly twice the number of calories. Which one do you think will leave you feeling full?

Figure 12   Food Labels of Food Items with a Low and High Diet Denominator

Nutrition Facts	
Serving Size 1 item 198g (198 g)	
Amount Per Serving	
Calories 404	Calories from Fat 122
	% Daily Value*
Total Fat 14g	21%
Saturated Fat 5g	24%
Trans Fat	
Cholesterol 18mg	6%
Sodium 1216mg	51%
Total Carbohydrate 55g	18%
Dietary Fiber 8g	31%
Sugars	
Protein 16g	
Vitamin A 3% • Vitamin C	0%
Calcium 23% • Iron	25%
*Percent Daily Values are based on a 2,000 calorie diet. Your daily values may be higher or lower depending on your calorie needs.	
©www.NutritionData.com	

Nutrition Facts	
Serving Size 1 item 99g (99 g)	
Amount Per Serving	
Calories 362	Calories from Fat 198
	% Daily Value*
Total Fat 22g	34%
Saturated Fat 5g	23%
Trans Fat	
Cholesterol 4mg	1%
Sodium 509mg	21%
Total Carbohydrate 36g	12%
Dietary Fiber 4g	15%
Sugars	
Protein 5g	
Vitamin A 0% • Vitamin C	0%
Calcium 9% • Iron	6%
*Percent Daily Values are based on a 2,000 calorie diet. Your daily values may be higher or lower depending on your calorie needs.	
©www.NutritionData.com	

Taco Bell™ bean burrito.   Taco Bell™ Nachos.

"Nutritional data and images courtesy of www.NutritionData.com."

Table 16   The Diet Denominator of Jersey Mike's™ Sandwiches

Mini Subs	Food Energy (Calories)	Weight (grams)	Diet Denominator
#7 Turkey Breast	210	233	0.90
#4 Cheese, Proscuittini, Cappacuolo	280	233	1.20
#2 Cheese, Ham, Cappacuolo	300	234	1.28
#6 Roast Beef	330	256	1.29
#18 Chicken Grilled (no mayo)	220	169	1.30
#3 Ham & Cheese	320	241	1.33
#11 Cheese, Ham, Salami	300	220	1.36
#1 BLT	250	182	1.37
#13 Jersey Mike's™ "Original" Cheese, Ham, Proscuittini, Cappacuolo, Salami, Pepperoni	390	276	1.41
#12 Cancro Special Cheese, Roast Beef, Pepperoni	400	262	1.53
#9 Club Supreme Roast Beef, Turkey, Swiss, Lettuce, Tomato, Mayo, Bacon	360	235	1.53
#8 Club Sub Cheese, Ham, Turkey, Lettuce, Tomato, Mayo, Bacon	350	228	1.54
#14 Vegetarian Swiss, Provolone, Lettuce, Tomatoes, Green Peppers, Onions	360	234	1.54
#18 Chicken breast parmesan (w/cheese & sauce)	350	190	1.84
#17 Jersey Mike's™ "Philly" Cheese Steak w/ Grilled Onions and Peppers	350	184	1.90
#20 Pastrami w/mustard	290	146	1.99
#10 Tuna	510	256	1.99
#19 Bar-B-Q Beef Sauce	320	159	2.01

Take home messages

- This plan will help you choose less energy dense foods even at fast food restaurants letting you eat more food volume while consuming fewer calories
- You will find great (energy lean) choices in the least suspecting places with this plan, it is up to you to choose the items you enjoy that are energy lean
- *The Diet Denominator* is not all about calories. Some choices might contain a few more calories; however, at the expense of a few more calories, some fast food choices will provide you with much more food leaving you feeling full
- Sandwiches make great (energy lean) choices with this plan. One of the best choices with this plan is Jersey Mike's™ turkey sandwich with a Diet Denominator of 0.9 while mashed potatoes from KFC™ make another good (energy lean) choice

Want to learn more? Many people believe that the secret to living a long life is plenty of exercise, rest, and eating well. But, what about eating less? Caloric restriction has been shown to increase lifespan in lower organisms. But will it work in humans? In an attempt to answer this question, researchers at Johns Hopkins University in Baltimore, Maryland, have undergone a long-term, 30% caloric restriction study using rhesus monkeys and squirrels. The study is still ongoing, but after 10 years the results seem to indicate that caloric restriction increases lifespan in both monkeys and squirrels (squirrels: six deaths in the control group vs. zero in the CR group and in the monkeys: six deaths in the control group vs. four in the caloric restriction group). Animals, much like humans die of a variety of illnesses as they age, which can often be affected by diet such as diabetes, cardiovascular disease, liver, and kidney disease. [20]

---

[20] Roth GS et al. Calorie restriction in primates: will it work and how will we know? *Journal of The American Geriatrics Society*. 1999;47:896-903.

11. How do everyday foods measure up to *The Diet Denominator*?

Most would agree that vegetables make great food choices for dieters and health conscious people alike. But with *The Diet Denominator*, you will learn that some choices are better than others and that they are not often obvious.

This chapter points out that some of the best foods on *The Diet Denominator* scale are pickles, lettuce, cabbage, asparagus, collards, and other vegetables with a high water content. Best of all, the choices on this plan are seemingly endless unlike most other diet plans. Thus, this plan does not restrict you or confine you or make use of unreasonable expectations. You will find that they can easily combine the calories from multiple ingredients in a meal and divide that by the combined value in grams and arise at *The Diet Denominator* for a meal or item made from various food items as illustrated in the table below.

Table 17   Calculating *The Diet Denominator*: Peanut Butter and Jelly Sandwich

Sandwich Item	Nutrition Facts	Diet Denominator
Jif Creamy Peanut Butter	190 calories per 32 grams	5.9
Grape Concord Jam	50 calories per 20 grams	2.5
Potato Bread	80 calories per 32 grams	2.5
Total	**320 calories per 84 grams**	3.8

This is also useful for foods from concentrate or that require milk such as cereal. For example, with the "Special K™" diet, there are 110 calories per serving in the plain cereal and 40 calories in the ½ cup of fat free milk. There are 31 grams in one serving of the cereal and ~120 mL (remember we will assume 1 mL equals 1 gram for our purposes). Therefore, 150 calories per 150 grams equals a Diet Denominator of 1.0, a good (energy lean) choice. *The Diet Denominator* of two common breakfast food choices are compared in Table 18 A and B below. As illustrated below, by choosing Quaker™ instant oatmeal, you are consuming a total of 286 grams (with water) and 170 calories. While Eggos™ are a good choice with the oatmeal you are eating 220 fewer calories yet 110 more grams. That said if you still choose the Eggos™, simply use lite syrup, which is a lower calorie alternative and you can reduce The Diet Denominator to below 3.0.

Table 18   Sample Breakfast Foods Choices

Description of Food	Food Energy (calories)	Weight (grams)	Diet Denominator
A. Quaker™ Instant Oatmeal (Cinnamon & Spice)	170 calories	46 grams plus 240 mL (grams) water	0.6 For oatmeal and added
B. Eggo's™ with Aunt Jemima's™ Original Syrup	180 calories plus 210 calories for 390 calories combined	70 grams plus 60 mL (grams) for 130 calories combined	3.0 For Eggo's and syrup

As described in the Chapter titled Satiety, one of the keys to volumetric (energy density) diets such is the fact that foods such as soups and stews have high water content; therefore, they make ideal food choices according to *The Diet Denominator*. In other words, *The Diet Denominator* even works with liquid foods like soup (but not drinks). Therefore, soup almost always makes a great (energy lean) choice with *The Diet Denominator*, which is important to keep in mind when making food choices. For example, Campbell's™ Beef Noodle Soup has 70 calories per 120 mL (grams) for a Diet Denominator of 0.6 and Campbell's™ Minestrone Soup has 90 calories per 120 mL (Grams) for a Diet Denominator of 0.8. For the purposes of this book, it is safe to assume that 1 mL of liquid equals 1 gram of food. Note: 1/2 cup equals 120 mL.

Did you know? Classic hummus, which is made largely from Chick peas, has 70 calories (50 from fat) per 28 grams, for a Diet Denominator of 2.5. Hummus is also high in fiber, making it a great food choice with this plan. Best of all, if purchased pre-made, simply serve and enjoy.

Other everyday foods measure up well with *The Diet Denominator*. For example, you will find that most produce such as fruits and vegetables are great with this plan. That is not surprising because these always make healthy alternatives that are easy to prepare, take with you if you are on the go, and best of all they taste great and many fruits even satisfy your sweet tooth.

Table 19   Diet Denominator of Some Fruits and Vegetables

Description of Food	Food Energy (calories)	Weight (grams)	Diet Denominator
Fruits			
Apples	53	110	0.5
Oranges	85	185	0.5
Pears	86	148	0.6
Vegetables			
Lettuce, green leaf, raw	5	36	0.1
Lettuce, iceberg, raw	10	72	0.1
Mixed vegetables, canned (corn, lima beans, peas, green beans, carrots)	67	182	0.4
Potato salad	357	250	1.4

The most popular cheese in America, thanks to pizza, is mozzarella, which has a Diet Denominator of around 2.8. It is not the cheese that makes pizza high in calories. Rather, the toppings, in particular, add significantly to the number of calories from pizza. Cheese is a good source of protein, which accounts to a significant proportion of the calories in many cheeses, which is better than calories from fat because protein helps to make you feel full and provides nutrients. An ounce of cheddar cheese contains seven times the protein of liquid milk. Much of the proteins in cheese are casein. The protein and moisture content in cheese varies widely by the variety and type of cheese, leading to large differences in *The Diet Denominator* ranging from around 2 -5 as illustrated in Table 20 below. Therefore, foods with protein such as cheese make great snacks.

Did you know? Hello Wisconsin! According to the United States Department of Agriculture, in 2008 the average American consumes more than 30 pounds of cheese, per person. It seems as though cheese has never before been available on so many dishes, in so many stores, or in so many varieties and people are gobbling it up.

Table 20   Diet Denominator of Various Cheeses

Description of Food	Food Energy (calories)	Weight (grams)	Diet Denominator
Parmesan cheese, grated	130	28.4	4.6
Cheddar cheese	115	28.4	4.1
Muenster cheese	105	28.4	3.7
Pasteurized processed cheese, American	105	28.4	3.7
Swiss cheese	105	28.4	3.7
Blue cheese	100	28.4	3.5
Provolone cheese	100	28.4	3.5
Pestered processed cheese, Swiss	95	28.4	3.4
Camembert cheese	115	38	3.0
Mozzarella cheese, whole milk	80	28.4	2.8

Take home messages

- Many everyday food items purchases at the grocery store and prepared at home make good food choices; however, *The Diet Denominator* is useful in helping you choose between food items thereby saving calories
- Some of the best foods on *The Diet Denominator* scale are pickles, lettuce, cabbage, asparagus, collards, and other vegetables with a high water content
- Foods such as soups and stews have low high water content; therefore, foods like soup and stews are ideal food choices according to *The Diet Denominator*
- For the purposes of this book, it is safe to assume that 1 mL of liquid equals 1 gram of food. Note: 1/2 cup equals 120 mL

Want to learn more? According to the American Institute for Cancer Research (AICR) report to the U.S. congress on the policy and action for cancer prevention, food, nutrition, and physical activity: a global perspective, it was stated that over 45% of colon cancer cases and 38% of breast cancer cases in the U.S. can be prevented by making changes in our diet, physical activity and weight control. This amounts to 49,000 fewer cases of colon cancer and 70,000 fewer cases of breast cancer each year. In fact, approximately one-third of the most common cancers can be prevented. The new WCRF/AICR Report is called Policy and Action for Cancer Prevention - Food, Nutrition, Physical Activity, and the Prevention of Cancer: a Global Perspective. For more information, visit the AICR's website available at: http://www.aicr.org/site/ and look for policy report.

12.   Empty calories and *The Diet Denominator*

What are empty calories? Empty calories usually refer to high energy (density) foods that are lacking the usual micronutrients and various other nutrients found in most other foods. Empty calories contain the same amount of energy (that can be converted to fat) as other food calories regardless of the source. The only difference is that empty calories do not provide other nutrients needed by the body. This is important in foods such as deep fried starches like French fries.

Other sources of empty calories are soda, candy, doughnuts, and other so-called junk foods. Alcohol is one of the greatest culprits as far as empty calories are concerned. Alcohol is not good for dieters for other reasons as well. Foods high in empty calories generally do not make you feel full compared to other foods; therefore, you are left wanting more and are more likely to consume more food later in that day.

> *Diet Denominator Facts:* Alcohol has 7 calories per gram; therefore, 1 gram alcohol contains 7 calories. Alcohol is one of the greatest culprits as far as empty calories are concerned. The average light beer contains a little over 100 calories per 12 ounce (355 mL) serving. While this amounts to a Diet Denominator of 0.3, liquids with alcohol cannot be compared with *The Diet Denominator*. This is, in part, because alcohol essentially contains nothing but empty calories. Alcohol decreases the metabolism of fat and adds to the negative effects on your caloric intake.

Examples of hidden (empty) calories include drinks such as sodas, energy drinks, juices, and coffee. There are 140 calories in a 12 ounce can of soda or a small soda at most fast food restaurants and the number of calories in a large or jumbo soda are even greater. A large, vanilla Iced Coffee from McDonalds™ has 270 calories, a large cappuccino has 290 calories, and a large, non-fat hot chocolate from McDonalds™ has a whopping 390 calories.

In addition to drinks, condiments are notorious culprits of hidden calories. For example, mayonnaise, ranch dressing, and even honey add a considerable number of calories to your food. In addition, sugars, milks, and half and half add numerous calories to drinks such as coffee.

Table 21 Diet Denominator of Some Common Condiments

Condiments	Calories	Grams	Diet Denominator
Hot Sauce	0	7	0.00
Mustard	0	12	0.00
Ketchup	10	9	1.11
Reduced Fat Sour Cream	30	21	1.43
Spicy Buffalo Sauce	70	43	1.63
Tangy Honey Mustard Sauce	70	43	1.63
Barbeque Sauce	50	28	1.79
Sweet 'N Sour Sauce	50	28	1.79
Hot Mustard Sauce	60	28	2.14
Spicy Avocado Ranch Dressing	110	35	3.14
Light Mayonnaise	40	12	3.33
Honey	50	14	3.57
Creamy Ranch Sauce	200	43	4.65
Mayonnaise	90	12	7.50

Did you know? Forbes.com makes a list of the most fattening drinks containing alcohol. They included the pina colada, margarita, long island ice tea, and white Russian. The Diet Denominator of pure alcohol (ethanol) is 0.78; therefore, The Diet Denominator does not work for alcohol, which is less dense than water. While trying to lose weight, the consumption of alcohol should be avoided. Otherwise, moderate alcohol consumption is acceptable.

Take home messages

- The term empty calories refers to high energy (density) foods that are lacking the usual micronutrients and various other nutrients found in most other foods
- Empty calories do not provide the nutrients needed by your body
- Foods high in empty calories included deep-fried foods, soda, candy, doughnuts, and other so-called junk foods

Want to learn more? Casual Drinking and Lipid Metabolism: Researchers say that a glass of wine a day may be beneficial to your health. But no matter how much you may want to believe it, it is not the alcohol that exerts this beneficial effect, rather, it is the phytochemicals such as resveratrol found in red wine in high concentrations. In a recent study at The University of California, Berkeley, researchers determined that the consumption of moderate levels (24 grams) of alcohol modestly activates lipogenesis or the production of fat. They also determined that the major end product of the alcohol consumed was acetate, but not fat. However, the acetate released by the liver traveled into the bloodstream where it inhibited lipolysis (breakdown of lipids) by 53% in peripheral tissues and a decrease in whole-body lipid oxidation in tissue such as muscle by 73%. Unfortunately, the study was only performed on 27 year-old healthy men who drink moderately. Additionally, the effects of alcohol on lipid metabolism, bodyweight, and body composition are complex so don't rule out the occasional nightcap just yet. [21]

---

[21] Scott Q Silver et al. American Journal of Clinical Nutrition. 1999;70:928-36.

13.   Understanding food labels and *The Diet Denominator*

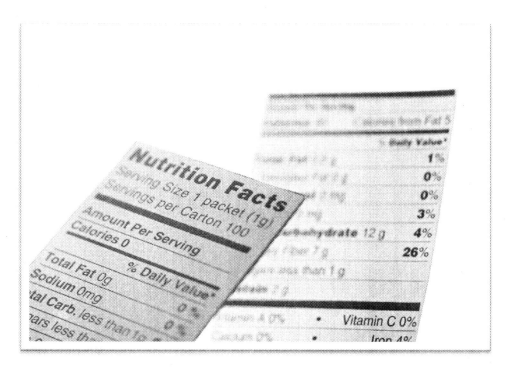

With *The Diet Denominator*, the only information on the food label that requires an understanding to begin using this plan is the calories per serving and the grams per serving. These two simple terms are easily located and clearly indicated on every food label by law.

In addition to the calories and grams in a serving, food labels contain a wealth of other important information. With a basic understanding of the nutrition facts that appear on all food labels, you can utilize this information to make informed food choices, which is an important part of learning how to maintain a healthy lifestyle and a balanced diet.

An ordinary food label contains information such as the number of calories from fat, total fat, saturated fat, and trans-fat to name a few. Here is an example of a food label from a slice of Domino's ultimate deep dish cheese pizza. You may have noticed that this label contains the % daily values for each of these nutrients. The % daily values appears on food labels and are important in helping you understand how much of a given nutrient a food item contains in relation to the recommended daily amount. Therefore, depending on the item, if the value is greater than 25-35% of the daily value, the item is relatively high in the item. This can be a good thing or a bad thing depending on the particular item.

For example, a food item with a greater proportion of fiber or a particular vitamin would be a good thing; however, a food item with a greater proportion of fat or cholesterol would be a bad thing. Figure 13 shows an ordinary food label from a pizza so that we can discuss daily values (DVs).

Figure 13   Domino's Ultimate Deep Dish Cheese Pizza

Nutrition Facts
Serving Size 1 slice 121g (121 g)

Amount Per Serving

Calories 332		Calories from Fat 113

	% Daily Value*
Total Fat 13g	19%
Saturated Fat 5g	24%
Trans Fat	
Cholesterol 17mg	6%
Sodium 679mg	28%
Total Carbohydrate 41g	14%
Dietary Fiber 3g	11%
Sugars 4g	
Protein 14g	

Vitamin A	8% •	Vitamin C	0%
Calcium	18% •	Iron	20%

*Percent Daily Values are based on a 2,000 calorie diet. Your daily values may be higher or lower depending on your calorie needs:

Calories		2,000	2,500
Total Fat	Less than	65g	80g
Sat Fat	Less than	20g	25g
Cholesterol	Less than	300mg	300mg
Sodium	Less than	2,400mg	2,400mg
Total Carbohydrate		300g	375g
Fiber		25g	30g

Calories per gram:
Fat 9   •   Carbohydrate 4   •   Protein 4

ⓒwww.NutritionData.com

The table below describes the typical items to understand on a food label. The %DV on any given food label is calculated by taking the amount of that item by the recommended daily value and multiplied by 100%. Using the example in Figure 13, one slice of pizza contains 13 grams of total fat and the recommended amount of fat is 65 grams of total fat per day. Therefore, 13/65 x 100% = 20%. It is important to note that these numbers are often rounded so these are not always exact but serve as a relatively reliable guide. For more information, visit the USDA's website, available at: http://www.nal.usda.gov/

Table 22   Food Components on an Ordinary Food Label*

Food Component	Recommended Daily Value**	Description
Total Fat	65 g (grams)	A macronutrient. Eating a low fat diet is recommended. Fat contains twice the amount of calories per gram than carbohydrates or protein.
Saturated Fat	20 g	The average American's diet is high in saturated fat and it should be reduced. This type of fat comes from animal sources.
Cholesterol	300 mg (milligrams)	A component of fat, particularly saturated fat.
Sodium	2,400 mg	A mineral and key **electrolyte**.
Potassium	3,500 mg	A mineral and key electrolyte.
Total Carbohydrate	300 g	Macronutrient made up of many sugars.
Dietary Fiber	25 g	A carbohydrate that is not well absorbed or not absorbed at all also called roughage as increases regularity.
Protein	50 g	A macronutrient. Composed of amino acids.
Vitamin A	5,000 IU (International Units)	Any of several related fat-soluble compounds having similar biological activity; best known for its importance for eyesight, tissues, bone, reproduction, and the immune system. Foods naturally high in this vitamin include liver, particularly of fish, egg yolks, and the fat component of dairy product.
Vitamin C	60 mg	Known as ascorbic acid, a water soluble vitamin naturally found in fruits and vegetables.
Calcium	1,000 mg	A mineral and key electrolyte.
Iron	18 mg	Mineral important in blood.
Vitamin D	400 IU	Foods naturally high in this vitamin include some fish liver oils, egg yolks, and fortified dairy products.
Vitamin E	30 IU	Foods naturally high in this vitamin include in wheat germ oil, cereal germs, egg yolk, liver, green plants, milk fat, and vegetable oils.
Vitamin K	80 µg (micrograms)	Important in the blood clotting process. Foods naturally high in this vitamin include green leafy

Food Component	Recommended Daily Value**	Description
		vegetables, liver, cheese, butter, and egg yolk.
Thiamin	1.5 mg	One of the B complex vitamins, which are water soluble. Foods naturally high in this vitamin include pork, organ meats, legumes, nuts, and whole grain or enriched cereals and breads.
Riboflavin	1.7 mg	One of the B complex, water soluble vitamins. Vitamin B2, important in numerous enzymes. Foods naturally high in this vitamin include milk, organ meats, eggs, leafy green vegetables, whole grains and enriched cereals and breads.
Niacin	20 mg	One of the B complex vitamins, which are water soluble. Also known as nicotinic acid or vitamin B3. Important in oxidation-reduction (redox) reactions.
Vitamin B6	2 mg	One of the B complex vitamins, which are water soluble. Important component of enzymes, nervous system function, and red blood cell function.
Folate (Folic acid)	400 µg	One of the B complex vitamins, which are water soluble. Important in DNA and amino acid metabolism.
Vitamin B12	6 µg	One of the B complex vitamins, which are water soluble. Deficiency in vitamin B12 is estimated to affect 10%-15% of individuals over the age of 60.
Biotin	300 µg	One of the B complex vitamins, which are water soluble. Important in many enzyme reactions.
Pantothenic acid (Vitamin B5)	10 mg	One of the B complex vitamins, which are water soluble. Important in many enzyme reactions.
Phosphorus	1,000 mg	Or phosphate is a mineral and key electrolyte.
Iodine	150 µg	A mineral. Found in iodized salt.
Magnesium	400 mg	A mineral and key electrolyte.
Zinc	15 mg	A mineral important to growth and development.
Selenium	70 µg	A mineral important in a variety of enzyme reactions.
Copper	2 mg	A mineral important in oxygen-reduction reactions.
Manganese	2 mg	A mineral important with **antioxidant** function.
Chromium	120 µg	A mineral important in glucose metabolism.
Molybdenum	75 µg	A mineral important in a variety of chemical reactions.
Chloride	3,400 mg	A mineral and key electrolyte.

*See Terms to Learn for more information. **Based on a 2000 calorie per day diet. For more information, visit the Linus Pauling Institute available at: http://lpi.oregonstate.edu/.

Diet Denominator Facts: One of the craziest diets that anyone has ever approached me about is the crushed ice diet. This is an extreme example of someone taking a scientific concept out of context. Crushed ice does require energy to melt. So logically you could burn energy (calories) by eating ice. The problem is that one food calorie is actually 1000 calories in scientific terms; therefore, the handful of calories that are required to melt ice in scientific terms is basically zero food calories. This misconception is because the term calorie, when used in science, in the discussion of chemical reactions such as melting ice, is only 1/1000 of a food calorie, which is insignificant in terms of your diet.

Take home messages

- DVs (Daily Values) are a new dietary reference term that appears on food labels. It is made up of two sets of references, DRVs and RDIs
- DRVs (Daily Reference Values) are a set of dietary references that applies to fat, saturated fat, cholesterol, carbohydrate, protein, fiber, sodium, and potassium
- RDIs (Reference Daily Intakes) are a set of dietary references based on the Recommended Dietary Allowances for essential vitamins and minerals and, in selected groups, protein

---

Want to learn more? There are two sets of reference values used in reporting nutrient information, Daily Reference values (DRVs) and Reference Daily Intakes (RDIs) based on specific reporting requirements. To avoid confusion, these values are combined to make up % daily values discussed in this chapter. For more information, visit U.S. Food and Drug Administration's, Center for Food and Safety and Applied Nutrition website, available at:

http://www.cfsan.fda.gov/list.html

---

14.   Keeping the Weight Off

Having read this book, you should be able to quickly and easily calculate *The Diet Denominator* of grocery store items, fast foods, and snack food items. You should be able to evaluate food choices time and time again across a variety of situations. Chapter by chapter, you will become more equipped with the tools you need to begin losing weight, the smart way, incrementally over time.

We all understand that losing weight is difficult. While this seems like an understatement, keeping the weight off is even more difficult. *The Diet Denominator* is not a fad. It is an educational diet plan that allows you to evaluate your food choices quickly and easily. As a result, you can consume fewer calories while consuming the same volume of food without feeling hungry. Once you have learned how to use *The Diet Denominator* as part of your everyday life, there is no reason you should stop using this plan. You will be able to make informed food choices quickly and easily as part of your daily routine.

With *The Diet Denominator*, keeping the weight off is easy because you are able to make informed food choices and choose foods that have a low energy density. One way to keep the weight off is to keep a diet journal. Diet journals (sometimes called diet records) are beneficial for a variety of reasons. Completing a diet journal is a form of self-monitoring, which, according to a variety of studies is proven to increase awareness, adherence, and positive results. By using any form of self-monitoring, you are more likely to succeed. Furthermore, diet journals allow you the time and means to recognize and reward yourself as you make progress towards your weight loss and eating goals, no matter how big or small the accomplishment. A sample weekly diet journal is located in Appendix 2.

With a diet journal, you can record your bodyweight, what you ate at each meal, the snacks you ate, and what and how often you chose to eat out. In addition, you can record foods with a good Diet Denominator that you enjoyed, and any other information related to your diet. You can record if you wanted to eat out but did not, or what foods you ate that you enjoyed and were good for you so you can eat again next time. Documenting you progress and choices is important because you may find you like certain foods that are healthy but just forget to purchase them or forget to choose them as part of your normal diet.

Poor diets are often due to convenience, not taste or for their ability to make us feel full. Therefore, the more often you can make a good food choice, the more routine that choice will become and the more weight you can lose. Diet journals allow you to determine your pitfalls and areas for improvement. In addition, weight loss is a slow and enduring battle that takes patience and persistence.

Dieting occurs incrementally over time, which is why this plan is great. It teaches you how to make informed food choices time and time again across a variety of situations. Change is difficult and hard to notice because it is often small and incremental. Thus the best way to notice incremental improvements in dieting habits and/or body weight changes might be to document those changes over time. Several online diet journals are available. These tools save time and make tracking results easier. They can make tracking changes enjoyable and interesting as the results continue to accumulate. Plus, many people find that it is fun to track their gains and even pitfalls so that they can learn a lot about their tendencies and keep focused on the bigger picture.

15.   Summary

What makes this plan so special is that it allows you to "fill your tank for less", meaning eating less energy dense foods leads to greater satiety. Importantly, this book is geared towards keeping the weight off. This is significant because the goal is to keep the weight off over the long-term.

The Diet Denominator is an educational diet plan that allows you to evaluate your food choices quickly and easily allowing you to consume fewer calories resulting in weight loss over time. Furthermore, this plan will teach you how to select energy lean food items time and time again helping you to make informed food choices quickly and easily at home, in the grocery store, even in a fast food restaurant.

Now that you have learned how to apply *The Diet Denominator* to your everyday life, there is no reason to stop using use this tool to make informed food choices quickly and easily anytime, anywhere.

The Diet Denominator is not just a diet plan, it is a life plan. *The Diet Denominator* is not just a tool it is a concept that applies to all situations, all foods, all people, and all types of meals. This plan is based on a fundamental principle of nutrition, energy density, which is comprised of the calorie and the gram. More specifically, *The Diet Denominator* is based on the energy density of foods (also known as volumetrics), which is a well tested and proven theory, but until now, lacked a system to use it. Volumetric diet plans require that you make knowledgeable food choices consisting of items that are energy lean, many of which make you feel full (increased satiety) and thus eat less afterwards. As illustrated in this book, you do not necessarily need to understand the energy density of foods to use this plan. That is because this plan uses a food evaluation tool that helps you to calculate the energy density of foods allowing you to choose the best food items quickly and easily. With *The Diet Denominator*, you determine if a food item is energy lean or energy dense. The more often you use this plan to assist you with choosing a meal, the better the plan will work and the sooner you can begin losing weight. Unlike calorie counting or other volumetric diet plans, this plan is simple to use and easy to apply to everyday life as it is not restricted to your home.

As you learned from reading this book, *The Diet Denominator* is not overly scientific and does not simply categorize foods as good carbohydrates versus bad, low protein versus high or by the number of calories it contains. This book utilizes a simple to use food evaluation tool that makes dieting simple, complete with real-world examples of foods you are already familiar with from fast food restaurants so that you can begin using this plan right away.

In conclusion, this book consists of a rewarding, fun, and easy to use food evaluation tool to help you make informed food choices in real time at home, in the grocery store, or even at fast food chains. Using this tool, choosing foods that are less energy dense is easy. This tool will allow you to consume fewer calories while feeling full without having to study which foods are energy lean or energy dense, and that is something that you can stick with, which is the key to keeping the weight off. In fact, you can select from any foods that they enjoy, so long as they are energy lean, based on *The Diet Denominator*.

This book demonstrates in simple terms how you can change your eating habits and make educated food choices quickly and easily in an effort to lose weight more easily and effectively while keeping the weight off. As a result, the reader will lose weight incrementally over time using a diet plan that they can stick to because they will not be left feeling hungry. Making informed food choices using this easy to use food evaluation tool is practical because it includes a Diet Denominator chart and journal that you can carry with you to help you make informed food choices quickly and easily as well as keep track of your progress.

Lastly, *The Diet Denominator* is not just a diet plan it is a life-plan that for just the cost of a book you can keep for life. Most importantly, successful dieting is about hope, faith, and conviction and it certainly is not easy. You should look within yourself for potential reasons for your bodyweight issues as often times there is an underlying issues and resolving those issues might make losing weight less difficult and more rewarding. Keep in mind, there is increasing evidence to suggest that people respond differently to dieting, genetics has an important role, and that your emotional status plays a critical role in your ability to lose weight. With any diet plan, after checking with your physician, it is important to increase your level of exercise to increase your chances of success and remember, you are in it for the long-haul so it is a marathon, not a sprint.

Appendix 1: Terms to Learn

Term to learn	Definition
Amino acids	Basic organic units that combine to form proteins. Amino acids are made up of hydrogen, carbon, oxygen, and nitrogen in the form of an "amino" ($-NH_2$) group.
Antioxidant	An enzyme or other organic substance, as vitamin E or beta carotene, that is capable of counteracting the damaging effects of oxidation in animal tissues.
Caloric content	The number of calories in a given amount of food
Calorie	A unit of measure pertaining to the amount of energy in food. Also known as large calorie, food calorie, or kilocalorie
Calories per gram	The number of food calories in one gram of a particular food item
Cholesterol	A sterol that occurs in animal tissues such as foods and in humans that is made in the body and comes from dietary sources; essential part of tissues and membranes and other molecules, however can be elevated in certain people
Diet Denominator	The number you select for a healthy diet with reduced calories/gram to help you lose weight
Dietary carbohydrates	Food component made up of multiple sugar molecules joined together. Also known as starches
Dietary fat	Food component made up of long-chain carbon units called fatty acids. Also known as lipids or oils
Dietary fiber	Non-starch polysaccharides and lignin that are not digested by enzymes in the small intestine. Also refers to as non-digestible carbohydrates of plant origin
Dietary proteins	Food component made up of amino acids and a major constituent of muscle
Electrolyte	Any of certain inorganic compounds, mainly sodium, potassium, magnesium, calcium, chloride, and bicarbonate, that dissociate in biological fluids into ions capable of conducting electrical currents and constituting a major force in controlling fluid balance within the body
Energy density	The amount of energy per unit of food. See calories per gram
Fluid ounce	Equals 30 mL
Fructose	A simple sugar primarily found in fruits and
Galactose	A simple sugar found in plants and animals and is less sweet than other sugars
Glucose	A cyclical, six-carbon sugar molecule (aldohexose) found as a free monosaccharide in fruits and other plants and in normal blood of all animals
Glycemic	The presence of glucose (sugar) in the blood
Glycemic index	A ranking of the rise in serum glucose that results from

Term to learn	Definition
	various food items
Grams	Equal to 0.035 ounces
Magic number	The average Diet Denominator of your ordinary diet
Mineral	A nonorganic homogeneous solid substance, usually a constituent of the earth's crust (i.e. iron)
Obesity	Obesity is a major public health problem and the leading nutritional disorder in the U.S. A widely accepted definition of obesity is body weight that is 20% or more in excess of ideal weight-for-height according to actuarial tables. By this definition, 34% of adults in the U.S. are obese, and there is evidence that the prevalence of obesity is increasing in both children and adults. The National Institutes of Health have defined obesity as a BMI of 30 or more, and overweight as a BMI between 25 and 30. By these criteria, 55% of adults are either overweight or obese
Ounce	Equal to 28 grams
Overweight	The National Institutes of Health have defined overweight as a BMI of 25.0-29.9
Saturated Fat	A fat, usually of animal origin, that is solid at room temperature of which the fatty acid chains cannot incorporate additional hydrogen atoms. An excess of these fats in the diet can raise cholesterol in the bloodstream
Sugars (simple sugars)	Refers to simple carbohydrates (monosaccharides and smaller oligosaccharides) with a chemical composition of $(C_6H_{12}O_6)n$ but often used to describe sucrose
Thermogenesis	Production of heat, by physiological processes
Unsaturated fat	Mono- or poly unsaturated fat refers to fat containing polyunsaturated fatty acids
Vitamin	Any of various organic substances that occur in many foods in small amounts and are necessary in trace amounts for the normal metabolic functioning of the body
Volumetrics	Any of a number of diet plans based on the energy density of foods, which leads to increased satiety and greater feeling of fullness

Appendix 2: Diet Denominator Tool

Step 1: Start here. Begin by finding the CALORIES of your food item from top to bottom.

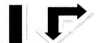

Step 2: Find the GRAMS from left to right across the page here.
The number at that intersection is The Diet Denominator.

	50	75	100	125	150	175	200	225	250
50	1	0.7	0.5	0.4	0.3	0.3	0.3	0.2	0.2
75	1.5	1	0.8	0.6	0.5	0.4	0.4	0.3	0.3
100	2	1.3	1	0.8	0.7	0.6	0.5	0.4	0.4
125	2.5	1.7	1.3	1	0.8	0.7	0.6	0.6	0.5
150	3	2	1.5	1.2	1	0.9	0.8	0.7	0.6
175	3.5	2.3	1.8	1.4	1.2	1	0.9	0.8	0.7
200	4	2.7	2	1.6	1.3	1.1	1	0.9	0.8
225	4.5	3	2.3	1.8	1.5	1.3	1.1	1	0.9
250	5	3.3	2.5	2	1.7	1.4	1.3	1.1	1
275	5.5	3.7	2.8	2.2	1.8	1.6	1.4	1.2	1.1
300	6	4	3	2.4	2	1.7	1.5	1.3	1.2
325	6.5	4.3	3.3	2.6	2.2	1.9	1.6	1.4	1.3
350	7	4.7	3.5	2.8	2.3	2	1.8	1.6	1.4
375	7.5	5	3.8	3	2.5	2.1	1.9	1.7	1.5
400	8	5.3	4	3.2	2.7	2.3	2	1.8	1.6
425	8.5	5.7	4.3	3.4	2.8	2.4	2.1	1.9	1.7
450	9	6	4.5	3.6	3	2.6	2.3	2	1.8
475	-	6.3	4.8	3.8	3.2	2.7	2.4	2.1	1.9
500	-	6.7	5	4	3.3	2.9	2.5	2.2	2
525	-	7	5.3	4.2	3.5	3	2.6	2.3	2.1
550	-	7.3	5.5	4.4	3.7	3.1	2.8	2.4	2.2
575	-	7.7	5.8	4.6	3.8	3.3	2.9	2.6	2.3
600	-	8	6	4.8	4	3.4	3	2.7	2.4
625	-	8.3	6.3	5	4.2	3.6	3.1	2.8	2.5
650	-	8.7	6.5	5.2	4.3	3.7	3.3	2.9	2.6
675	-	9	6.8	5.4	4.5	3.9	3.4	3	2.7
700	-	-	7	5.6	4.7	4	3.5	3.1	2.8

Step 1: Start here. Begin by finding the CALORIES of your food item from top to bottom.
Step 2: Find the GRAMS from left to right across the page here.
The number at that intersection is The Diet Denominator.

	275	300	325	350	375	400	425	450	475
50	0.2	0.2	0.2	0.1	0.1	0.1	0.1	0.1	0.1
75	0.3	0.3	0.2	0.2	0.2	0.2	0.2	0.2	0.2
100	0.4	0.3	0.3	0.3	0.3	0.3	0.2	0.2	0.2
125	0.5	0.4	0.4	0.4	0.3	0.3	0.3	0.3	0.3
150	0.5	0.5	0.5	0.4	0.4	0.4	0.4	0.3	0.3
175	0.6	0.6	0.5	0.5	0.5	0.4	0.4	0.4	0.4
200	0.7	0.7	0.6	0.6	0.5	0.5	0.5	0.4	0.4
225	0.8	0.8	0.7	0.6	0.6	0.6	0.5	0.5	0.5
250	0.9	0.8	0.8	0.7	0.7	0.6	0.6	0.6	0.5
275	1	0.9	0.8	0.8	0.7	0.7	0.6	0.6	0.6
300	1.1	1	0.9	0.9	0.8	0.8	0.7	0.7	0.6
325	1.2	1.1	1	0.9	0.9	0.8	0.8	0.7	0.7
350	1.3	1.2	1.1	1	0.9	0.9	0.8	0.8	0.7
375	1.4	1.3	1.2	1.1	1	0.9	0.9	0.8	0.8
400	1.5	1.3	1.2	1.1	1.1	1	0.9	0.9	0.8
425	1.5	1.4	1.3	1.2	1.1	1.1	1	0.9	0.9
450	1.6	1.5	1.4	1.3	1.2	1.1	1.1	1	0.9
475	1.7	1.6	1.5	1.4	1.3	1.2	1.1	1.1	1
500	1.8	1.7	1.5	1.4	1.3	1.3	1.2	1.1	1.1
525	1.9	1.8	1.6	1.5	1.4	1.3	1.2	1.2	1.1
550	2	1.8	1.7	1.6	1.5	1.4	1.3	1.2	1.2
575	2.1	1.9	1.8	1.6	1.5	1.4	1.4	1.3	1.2
600	2.2	2	1.8	1.7	1.6	1.5	1.4	1.3	1.3
625	2.3	2.1	1.9	1.8	1.7	1.6	1.5	1.4	1.3
650	2.4	2.2	2	1.9	1.7	1.6	1.5	1.4	1.4
675	2.5	2.3	2.1	1.9	1.8	1.7	1.6	1.5	1.4
700	2.5	2.3	2.2	2	1.9	1.8	1.6	1.6	1.5

Appendix 3: Diet Denominator of Some Common Food Items

Food Item	Calories	Grams	Diet Denominator
Corn oil	125	14	8.90
Lamb, chops, lean	135	48	2.9
Trout, broiled, with butter	175	85	2.06
Haddock, breaded, fried	175	85	2.06
Pancakes, buckwheat, from mix	55	27	2.04
Eggs, cooked, fried	90	46	1.96
Tuna, canned, drained, oil, chuck light	165	85	1.94
Chicken a la king, home recipe	470	245	1.92
Lamb, leg, roasted, lean only	140	73	1.92
Turkey, roasted, dark meat	160	85	1.88
Tuna salad	375	205	1.83
Beef roast, eye o round, lean	135	75	1.80
Chicken, stewed, light and dark meat	250	140	1.79
Turkey, roasted, light and dark meat	145	85	1.71
Chicken, roasted, drumstick	75	44	1.70
Miso soup	470	276	1.70
Eggs, cooked, scrambled/omelet	100	61	1.64
Turkey, roasted, light meat	135	85	1.59
Pork, cured, ham, roasted, lean	105	68	1.54
Chicken and noodles, home coked	365	240	1.52
Vienna sausage	45	16	1.5
Pinto beans, dry, cooked, drained	265	180	1.47
Macaroni, cooked, firm	190	130	1.46
Potato salad made with mayo	360	250	1.44
Sweet potatoes, candied	145	105	1.38
Spaghetti and meatballs with sauce	330	248	1.33
Potatoes, au gratin, home cooked	325	245	1.33
Rice, brown, cooked	230	195	1.18
Tapioca pudding from mix	145	130	1.12
Macaroni, cooked	155	140	1.11
Rice, white, cooked	225	205	1.10
Potatoes, baked with skin	220	202	1.09
Potatoes, mashed, recipe	225	210	1.07
Raspberries, frozen, sweetened	255	250	1.02
Chicken chow mein, home recipe	255	250	1.02
Sweet potatoes, canned, mashed	260	255	1.02
Refried beans, canned	295	290	1.02

Food Item	Calories	Grams	Diet Denominator
Strawberries, frozen, sweetened	275	284	0.97
Macaroni and cheese, canned	230	240	0.96
Banana	105	114	0.92
Cottage cheese, low fat 2%	205	226	0.91
Beef and vegetable stew, home recipe	220	245	0.90
Apricot, canned, heavy syrup	215	258	0.83
Cream of mushroom soup with milk, canned	205	248	0.83
Cream of chicken soup with milk, canned	190	248	0.77
Applesauce, canned, sweetened	195	255	0.76
Pears, canned, heavy syrup	190	255	0.75
Fruit cocktail, canned, heavy syrup	185	255	0.73
Cream of wheat, mix n eat	100	142	0.70
Yogurt, with low fat milk, plain	145	227	0.64
tangerines, canned, light syrup	155	252	0.62
Pineapple, canned, juice pack	35	58	0.60
Kiwifruit, raw	45	76	0.59
Grapefruit, canned, syrup pack	150	254	0.59
Apples, raw, unpeeled, 3 per lb	80	138	0.58
Cream of wheat	140	244	0.57
Blueberries, raw	80	145	0.55
Yogurt, with nonfat milk	125	227	0.55
Cream of mushroom soup with water	130	244	0.53
Pears, canned, juice pack	125	248	0.50
Raspberries, raw	60	123	0.49
Pineapples, raw, diced	75	155	0.48
Oranges, raw, sectioned	85	180	0.47
Apricots, raw	50	106	0.47
Cream of chicken soup with water	115	244	0.47
Artichokes, globe, cooked, drained	55	120	0.46
Peaches, raw, sliced	75	170	0.44
Applesauce, canned, unsweetened	105	244	0.43
Tangerines, raw	35	84	0.42
Carrots, raw, whole	30	72	0.42
Peaches, raw	35	87	0.40
Chicken chow mein, canned	95	250	0.38
Beef noodle soup, canned	85	244	0.35

Food Item	Calories	Grams	Diet Denominator
Grapefruit, raw, pink	40	120	0.33
Minestrone soup, canned	80	241	0.33
Vegetable beef soup, canned	80	244	0.33
watermelon, raw	155	482	0.32
Chicken noodle soup, canned	75	241	0.31
Strawberries, raw	45	149	0.30
Vegetarian soup, canned	70	241	0.29
Broccoli, raw	40	151	0.26
Mushrooms, cooked, drained	40	156	0.26
Cauliflower, raw	25	100	0.25
Asparagus	15	60	0.25
Chicken rice soup, canned	60	241	0.25
Spinach, cooked from raw, drained	40	180	0.22
Lettuce, loose leaf	10	56	0.18
Cucumbers	5	28	0.18
Celery, raw	20	120	0.17

Appendix 4: Diet Denominator of your Favorite Foods

Food Item	Calories	Grams	Diet Denominator
Example: refried beans, canned	*217*	*238*	*0.9*
1.			
2.			
3.			
4.			
5.			
6.			
7.			
8.			
9.			
10.			

Appendix 5: Weekly Diet Journal

Day	Breakfast	Lunch	Dinner	Snacks	Weight	Exercise
Monday						
Tuesday						
Wednesday						
Thursday						
Friday						
Saturday						
Sunday						